Psychotropic Drugs in Psychiatry

Michael Shepherd, M.D.

JASON ARONSON
NEW YORK • LONDON

For M.H.
Gradu diverso, una via

ISBN: 0-87668-273-5

Library of Congress Catalog Number: 81-66758

10 9 8 7 6 5 4 3 2 1

Manufactured in the United States of America

Contents

Preface

The treatment of mental illness was revolutionized in the early 1950s by the introduction of a variety of new drugs. The arrival of these compounds, which included meprobamate, chlorpromazine, hydroxyzine, benactyzine, and reserpine, opened a new chapter in the history of chemotherapy and catalyzed a remarkable burst of interest and inquiry by both clinical psychiatrists and nonmedical scientists. Until this time the links between pharmacology and psychiatry had been more dependent on the enthusiasm and interest of individual workers than on a general acknowledgment of the need to explore common ground. Within a few years the situation was transformed. An old word, psychopharmacology, was rediscovered and generally accepted as the term of choice for a large, federated area of activity involving several related biological and behavioral sciences. By the end of the decade J. D. French was able to say that psychopharmacology had generated "an illuminating flash of brilliance, a promising excavation into the mountain of ignorance and an exceptionally large amount of flying rubble."

Today the gains already associated with the establishment of psychopharmacology can be put in perspective. Research workers have provided advances in knowledge about such diverse topics as receptor theory, central neurotransmission, and animal behavior. Clinical innovations have been made in the rational treatment of Parkinson's disease and in the more effective symptomatic management in major and minor mental illnesses. Nonetheless, the gap between clinical knowledge and scientific understanding remains so uncomfortably wide that the research-minded physician is constantly stimulated to reexamine assumptions concerning the etiology and outcome of the disorders that he treats in relation to an ever increasing quantity of new information. At the same time, as a prescriber of psychotropic drugs, he also has to be aware of the wider social and economic implications of this form of medication for the community at large.

The chapters included in this volume reflect some of the ways in which psychopharmacology has impinged on the perspectives of clinical psychiatry. The material was selected from papers written over a period of twenty years. During this time it has been possible to delineate three broad categories of inquiry, all of which have engaged my personal involvement and constitute the logical basis of each of the three sections in the book. In the first section I focus on the drugs themselves, survey the problem of their classification, and illustrate some of the basic clinical and pharmacological issues by referring to particular examples. The second section concentrates on the central topic of therapeutic evaluation, with special attention paid to the design of clinical experiments and to the interaction of nonpharmacodynamic factors with drug interaction. In the third section I examine some of the wider social implications of prescribing psychotropic medication for both the mentally ill and the population at large.

These broad topics are introduced and succeeded by two essays that provide a general framework for a wide-ranging collection of contributions to an important field of scientific research and clinical practice. Taken together, they demonstrate clearly the widespread ramifications of modern pharmacotherapeutics in the mental health field.

Acknowledgments

The author wishes to thank the publishers of the following journals and books for permission to reprint material in this volume:

Progress and problems in mental health. In Taylor, D. (Ed.) *Benefits and Risks in Medical Care.* London: Office of Health Economics, 1974.

The classification of psychotropic drugs. *Psychological Medicine,* 1972, 2(2):96–110.

Reserpine: Problems associated with the use of a so-called "tranquilizing agent." *Proceedings of the Royal Society of Medicine,* 1956, 49(10):849.

The benzodiazepines. *Prescribers' Journal,* 1972, 12(6):144.

Centrally acting drugs. In *Evaluation of New Drugs in Man: Proceedings of the Second International Pharmacological Meeting.* New York: Pergamon Press, 1965.

Interaction between centrally-acting drugs in man: Some general considerations. *Proceedings of the Royal Society of Medicine,* 1965,58:964.

The evaluation of treatment in psychiatry. In Sainsbury, P. and Kreitman, N. (Eds.), *Methods of Psychiatric Research.* London: Oxford University Press, 1975.

Comparative psychiatric treatment in different countries. In Richter, D., Tanner, J. M., Lord Taylor and Zangwill, O. L. (Eds.), *Aspects of Psychiatric Research.* London: Oxford University Press, 1962.

Therapeutic problems with psychotropic drugs: Some epidemiological considerations. *Psychiatria, Neurologia, Neurochirugia,* 1969, 72:503–506.

Impact of long-term neuroleptics on the community: Advantages and disadvantages (with D. C. Watt). In Boissier, J. R., Hippius, H., and Pichot, P. (Eds.), *Neuropsychopharmacology.* New York: Elsevier, 1975.

Clinical and social factors relevant to outcome. In Nuffield Provincial Hospitals Trust, *The Epidemiology of Mental Illness: A Symposium,* London: Oxford University Press, 1962.

Research in the field of psychiatry. *British Medical Journal,* 1969, 4:161.

The influence of specific and non-specific factors on the clinical effects of psychotropic drugs. In Rothlin, E. (Ed.), *Neuropsychopharmacology, Volume Two.* New York: Elsevier 1961.

The effectiveness of drugs in relationship to psychological and social forms of treatment. In Bradley, P. B., Flugel, F., and Hoch, P. (Eds.). *Neuropsychopharmacology, Volume Three.* New York: Elsevier, 1964.

Clinical trials: A personal view. *British Medical Journal,* 1971, 1:457.

The method of the multi-centred clinical trial. In Brill, H., Cole, J. O., Deniker, P., Hippius, H., and Bradley, P. B. (Eds.), *Neuropsychopharmacology.* New York: Elsevier, 1968.

Evaluation of psychotropic drugs in the treatment of depression: 1959–1969. In Harris, E. L. and Fitzgerald, J. D. (Eds.), *The Principles and Practice of Clinical Trials.* London: Livingstone, 1970.

Continuation treatment with antidepressant medication. In Bohaček, N. (Ed.), *Psihofarmakologija 3.* Zagreb, Yugoslavia: Medicinska Naklada, 1974.

The use and abuses of drugs in psychiatry. *Lancet,* 1970, 1:31–33.

Prologue

Chapter 1

A View in Retrospect

It is now generally accepted that the widespread use of psychotropic medication has been the most obvious single change in the treatment of mental disorders in the postwar period. Any attempt at evaluation of such treatment, however, must take into account several related factors. In the first place, treatment in psychiatry is traditionally a triadic procedure including psychological measures and social or environmental manipulation, as well as the use of physical agents. The lineage of the psychological approach can be traced to the "moral" forms of treatment in the nineteenth century and to Pinel's emphasis on the significance of "consolatory language, kind treatment and the revival of extinguished hopes" in treating the mentally disturbed. The social aspects of treatment are omnipresent, since they determine not only the structure of psychiatric services but provide close links with the matrix of public and professional opinion, on which all forms of psychiatric intervention depend. Psychotropic drugs, of course, fall into the category of physical agents, but it is important to recall that their arrival radically altered the concept of the physical dimension of psychiatric treatment. If, for example, one looks at the first edition of so influential a book as Sargant and Slater's *An Introduction to Physical Methods of Treatment in Psychiatry,* originally published in 1944, there are full chapters on 'the insulin treatment of schizophrenia; modified insulin therapy; convulsion therapy; continuous sleep treatment; diet, vitamins and endocrines; prefrontal leucotomy; and the malarial treatment of general paralysis. By contrast, apart from some discussion of the special uses of intravenous barbiturates and the anticonvulsants then available, reference to drugs is compressed into the single chapter on chemical sedation and stimulation, in which the substances considered are bromides, paraldehyde, barbiturates, amphetamine sulfate, and thyroid preparations.

Against this background, the course of events following the arrival of the first wave of psychotropic drugs in the early 1950s can be broadly divided into three phases. There was, of course, some overlapping in the time and substance of these three, but for convenience, the first phase can be regarded as having extended through the 1950s, the second phase as having lasted until the late 1960s, and the third phase as existing up to the present. I entitle them the phases of initial impact, evaluation, and consolidation, respectively, and propose to consider each in turn.

PHASE 1: INITIAL IMPACT

The phenothiazines, reserpine, the butyrophenones, the monoamine oxidase inhibitors, the tricyclic compounds, the propanediols and the thioxanthenes all became available within a short span of time. The most obvious consequence of their introduction into clinical practice was the speed and completeness with which they were adopted. Indeed, within a few years the staple treatment of the functional psychoses had been transformed; insulin units had closed down in most hospitals and there was a sharp decline in the frequency of the other crude forms of physical treatment, including electroconvulsive therapy. In office practice, too, the newer drugs rapidly superseded their predecessors.

The spirit of acceptance was of course not universal, and several studies showed that the expressed attitudes of psychiatrists to the three broad modalities of treatment influenced their opinions of pharmacotherapy (Shepherd 1964). Some of the opposition was voiced by proponents of psychological treatment, on the grounds that an impersonal prescription was no substitute for the doctor-patient relationship. This viewpoint, that of the committed psychotherapist, has in fact remained consistent to the present. It was recently stated clearly by a prominent American psychoanalyst, in a contribution to the current debate on the declining prestige of psychoanalysis in the United States. Asked her opinion of drug therapy, she said: "I think that drug therapy is like a crutch. It can help to tune down panic states and severe anxiety states for the moment, but I don't think that it has any lasting effects. Psychoanalysis really tries to treat the motives and causes of these anxieties. The patient needs some meditative process: What is it all about? he must ask, and how am I my own worst enemy? Drugs cannot eliminate alienation, mistrust and fear" (Weigert 1973).

The initial reaction of several advocates of social psychiatry to chemotherapy was also guarded, especially with regard to the controversial issue of the resident populations of mental hospitals, which began to decline in the mid-1950s after having risen steadily for many years. The role played by drugs in this trend was contested in the United Kingdom by Sir Aubrey Lewis, who put the issue bluntly: "If we had to choose between abandoning the use of all the new psychotropic drugs and abandoning the Industrial Resettlement Units and other social facilities available to us, there would be no hesitation about the choice: the drugs would go" (Lewis 1959). On the same lines, Ödegaard (1964) in Norway pointed to the variation between statistics from different institutions and concluded, paradoxically, that "in hospitals with a favorable therapeutic situation the psychotropic drugs brought little or no improvement in the rate of discharges. In hospitals with a low pre-drug discharge rate on the other hand, the improvement was considerable."

Despite these factional disagreements, however, the vast majority of psychiatrists welcomed and adopted the new array of psychotropic drugs in their clinical practice. Furthermore, the scientific significance of the new drugs was acknowledged by the need to resurrect an old term, *psychopharmacology,* to define the new scientific discipline they created. It must be emphasized, however, that the psychopharmacologists did not provide a more rational understanding for the basis of the treatment methods they used. Most of the drugs were introduced and used empirically, and neither their site nor their mode of action was clearly understood. Reviewing the accumulated experimental work of the period I was forced to conclude that "while a great deal of knowledge has accrued about the hungry pigeon, the thirsty rat, and the frightened monkey, relatively few attempts have been made to determine whether the information can be applied to human responses" (Shepherd 1961b).

Perhaps more surprising during this phase was the relative lack of clinical research designed to evaluate the efficacy of pharmacological treatment. Most of the extravagant claims made on behalf of individual drugs were unrelated to controlled experimentation. In consequence, the verdict I felt compelled to express on the status of psychopharmacology in 1960 was understandably cautious.

"In the light of current knowledge, it would be difficult . . . to base the reputation of psychopharmacology on a large body of established knowledge about either the therapeutic value or the pharmacodynamic action of the psychotropic drugs. To what then can the high status of the subject be attributed? Though it may not be possible yet to provide a comprehensive answer to this question it is apparent that a full explanation does not fall within the framework of the physical or clinical sciences. Status, we may recall, is a sociologic concept closely related to economic class, and the evidence supports Professor Toman's view that it has been the socioeconomic impact of new drugs in psychiatry which has inspired the 'veritable explosion of research on the action of drugs.' For 150 years the history of the therapeutics of mental disorder has demonstrated the importance of social and professional attitudes as the pendulum has oscillated between the 'moral' and the so-called physical methods of treatment. In retrospect it is clear that the newer pharmacologic compounds were introduced to psychiatry at a time which favored their adoption: on the one hand, a growing disillusion with psychological treatment had become increasingly evident even where these methods had been taken up with most enthusiasm; on the other, the seams of the older physical method of treatment had been exhausted and even their most ardent advocates were dissatisfied with the crudity of the empirical tools at their disposal. The great majority of eclectic psychiatrists had long recognized the limitations of available methods of treatment and they have welcomed the clinical possibilities of the new drugs, finding great advantages in the relative flexibility of pharmacotherapy and, less obviously, in the employment of measures which are more in keeping with the traditional forms of medical care. Their eagerness to employ pharmacologic methods of treatment, stimulated by a vigorous campaign on the part of the pharmaceutical industry, has played an important role in the widespread adoption of drug therapy in psychiatric institutions. The still more extensive use of drugs in the extramural practice of psychiatrists and general practitioners appears to reflect not only the attitudes and habits of physicians but also the expectation of their patients as representatives of a public alive to the importance of mental distress and strongly influenced by the cult of tranquility. . . .

"Nonetheless, while the rise of psychopharmacology carries lessons for the medical sociologist, an interdisciplinary scientific program of great potential value has been evolved. Whatever the practical outcome of the effort which is being expended on the pharmacotherapy of neuropsychiatric disorders, it is certain that the interest of distinguished workers in many fields has been aroused and encouraged by the preliminary findings. Their work signifies aspiration rather than achievement at the present time, but the assurance of their prospective collaboration justifies a sober optimism for the future" (Shepherd 1961b).

PHASE 2: EVALUATION

There were several productive developments of the evaluation phase. With the significant exception of the beta-adrenergic blockers and benzodiazepines for the treatment of anxiety, few radically new compounds were introduced during this time; but numerous modifications of established psychotropic drugs made their appearance. Some of the potential hazards as well as the advantages of psychotropic medication also became more apparent, in the form of a host of recorded adverse reactions (Shepherd et al. 1968). It was, indeed, one such phenomenon—the hypertensive crises associated with the interaction of monoamine oxidase inhibitors with various foodstuffs—which furnished a particularly elegant demonstration of how parallel animal and human studies could be applied productively to a problem of clinical psychopharmacology (Blackwell and Marley 1966). During this time too, the implications of psychotropic drug action as a research tool for studying the biological mechanisms of mental illness were underlined in a 1967 World Health Organization Scientific Group report. Also significantly, the first textbook of psychopharmacology, coauthored by a psychiatrist, a clinical pharmacologist, and a biochemist, appeared at about the same time (Shepherd et al. 1968).

With further clinical experience the more extreme biases for and against pharmacotherapy were tempered by a growing appreciation of its value and limitations. If it became apparent that the control of symptoms was a more realistic objective for psychopharmacology than the cure of disease, it was clear also that this achievement had helped facilitate the changing climate of opinion toward mental disorder embodied in the United Kingdom's Mental Health Act of 1959. Indeed, the result was singled out for comment by the Chief Medical Officer of Great Britain's Department of Health and Social Security: "More active psychiatric treatment made more effective by the development of new drugs and greater understanding of the social problems by the general public as well as by those professionally concerned, has radically altered the position of the mentally ill" (Godber 1973). Insofar as this view is based on the increasing number of patients discharged from mental hospitals, however, it implies the existence of extramural facilities, which cannot always be taken for granted.

In many ways the most far-reaching step at this time, however, was the increasing recognition of the need for clinical evaluation of psychotropic medication, while also taking into account the role played by the biologically "nonspecific," (i.e., psychosocial) aspects of psychotropic chemotherapy (Shepherd 1961a). It was soon demonstrated, for example, that the pharmacodynamic action of the psychotropic drugs could not account for more than about one-third of the observed improvement in an institutionalized psychiatric population, and that the nonspecific factors must claim attention in any attempt to evaluate the observed effects. These nonspecific factors made it very difficult to interpret the results of many of the early hospital reports, which were for the most part conducted on a small scale. The difficulties were increased in the treatment of outpatient, or "minor," emotional disorders, which are influenced still more profoundly by psychological and social factors.

Probably the most impressive demonstration of the issue of specific versus nonspecific factors was provided by the large-scale, multicenter clinical trial of the treatment of depressive illness, conducted under the aegis of a Medical Research Council subcommittee concerned with clinical trials of various therapies. The need for such an investigation was at the time pressing, as there were already several conflicting reports about the value of antidepressant drugs (Kimbell et al. 1965). The objective of the study was to compare the efficacy of electroconvulsive therapy, a tricyclic compound, a monoamine oxidase inhibitor, and a placebo in the treatment of inpatients suffering from depressive disorders. The drugs and placebo were administered by the double-blind method and progress was assessed by a standardized procedure. Uniform criteria were established for admission to and exclusion from the study, so as to ensure as much homogeneity as possible. Fifty-five physicians working in some thirty hospitals provided more than 250 patients. All were followed up for six months from the date of entry into the trial, receiving their treatment in hospital for the first month and, on their discharge, visiting the outpatient department at specified intervals.

Two conclusions drawn from this investigation may be emphasized. First, its successful prosecution proved that a complex, multicenter trial, along lines which the Medical Research Council had pioneered in other branches of medicine, could be successfully applied to psychiatry. Second, while about one-third of the patients receiving the placebo responded satisfactorily, there proved to be no way of distinguishing the effects of drug from placebo in patients who responded to both. Therefore, although the drugs were being misused (in the sense of being used unnecessarily by a substantial section of the trial population), the information obtained in the trial was of only limited value to the clinician charged with the care of individuals.

PHASE 3: CONSOLIDATION

The psychopharmacological developments of the past few years may briefly be categorized as scientific, clinical, and social.

On the scientific front, technical advances have stimulated an interest in psychotropic drugs among clinical pharmacologists, and there has been a welcome and productive increase in the number and quality of collaborative studies between laboratory and clinical workers. It is now evident that the current intensive study of the role of the biogenic amines in neurotransmission was greatly stimulated by study of the biological action of psychotropic compounds. Furthermore, although such work has led to no therapeutic advance against mental disorders comparable to that derived from the use of L-dopa in Parkinsonism, it has facilitated derivation of a number of sophisticated biological hypotheses from animal studies testable in man. One such hypothesis, for example, is that the phenothiazines and the butyrophenones act by increasing catecholamine turnover through a feedback mechanism consequent on their blocking action on postsynaptic receptors. On this assumption it was postulated that after a-methyltyrosine inhibition of tyrosine hydroxylase, there would be potentiation of the action of these drugs. Carlsson and his colleagues have shown this to be true, not only in studies with food-reinforced operant behavior in rats, but also in the treatment of schizophrenic symptomatology in humans (Carlsson et el. 1972).

In the clinical field a new crop of "me-too" compounds has arrived along with a tendency to explore drug combinations and to employ them in conjunction with other forms of treatment. More important, the concept of drug evaluation has been extended not only to the question of whether the drug is effective, but also, to the questions of for whom it is effective for and for how long it should be prescribed. The first of these latter two questions, involving as it does the attempt to identify drug responders, has received an impetus from methods developed to estimate plasma levels of several psychotropic compounds (Drug and Therapeutics Bulletin 1974), although so far the results of these studies have been equivocal with respect to both therapeutic response and adverse effects. The question of length of prescription entails a more complex view of drug evaluation, one directly relevant to two major chemotherapeutic innovations in the management of psychotic illness. In the continued absence of superior new compounds these two are: (1) the controversial use of lithium carbonate as a "prophylactic" agent in the treatment of recurrent affective illness (Blackwell and Shepherd 1968), and (2) the use of long-acting phenothiazines for schizophrenia (Shepherd and Watt 1975). So-called maintenance therapy, which has been advocated as an essential feature of both these regimens, calls for a clinical assessment that takes into account the time-scale on which both are administered; several studies have been designed with this objective (Hirsch et al. 1973, Mindham et al. 1973).

The most striking recent social trend in psychopharmacology has been the remarkable increase in prescriptions of the benzodiazepines. While Parish has documented this phenomenon in the United Kingdom, Blackwell (1973) has recently pointed to a parallel situation in the United States, especially concerning diazepam. As he goes on to show, only about 30 percent of the use of diazepam has been for mental illness: 17 percent has been for musculoskeletal, 16 percent for circulatory, 8 percent for geriatric, 6 percent for neurological, 6 percent for gastrointestinal, and 3 percent for genitourinary illnesses; 7 percent has been for a miscellany of other conditions. Furthermore, in nearly two thirds of cases diazepam has been prescribed in combination with other substances. Clearly, therefore, the so-called anxiolytic drugs are being widely used in medicine by a variety of specialists for a variety of conditions.

What is the explanation for this remarkable phenomenon? One observer has stressed the role of the pharmaceutical industry. Another commentator is on record as having stated that "we must view the present volume of use of psychotropic medicines in much the same light as we should view the amount of claret and port consumed by the Victorian middle-classes" (Teeling-Smith 1973). This argues that the lowering of class barriers has democratized the form—if not the content—of drug-taking behavior. Other observers accuse the medical profession of overprescription or invoke the vagaries of fashion. To add to the miscellany I would recall John Ryle's comment on the treatment of minor emotional disorders, written some thirty years ago:

> Faults of upbringing, domestic stress, industrial fatigue, inadequate sleep and holidays, economic anxieties—factors eventually alterable by improved education, more ample accommodation for families, factory welfare and social insurance—have also played their significant part. In the meantime we try to cope with their consequences with bottles of medicine and certificates and a multiplication of psychiatric clinics at an ever-increasing cost to the community.

Since opinions far outnumber facts in so nebulous an area as overprescription, we should be grateful to the state of South Carolina, which recently banned benzodiazepines from its Medicaid program on the grounds of expense (Keller and McCurdy unpublished). A comparison of prescription-writing six months before and after the ban showed that 35 percent of prescriptions in the original sample were accounted for by phenothiazines, antidepressants, and barbiturates, but that 65 percent of drugs were not replaced after the ban. There are, of course, several possible explanations: for example, the banned drugs may have been obtained privately or self-medication may have increased.

Certainly the drug-use figures we have are large enough to direct attention to the abuse-potential of many psychotropic drugs. Here it is relevant to recall (1) that the 1971 Vienna Convention on Psychotropic Drugs required the World Health Organization to supply an assessment of these substances, and (2) that there is an increasing shift of emphasis from physical to what is now called psychic dependence on psychotropic drugs; this dependence has been described as "characterized by mainly psychic or mental phenomena on prolonged intake, such as drug-seeking behavior, an intensive 'liking' for the drug, and an overpowering compulsion or drive to continue to take the drug to achieve a different state of mind, with less obvious symptoms on withdrawal, the prolonged use in a number of cases leading to unsocial behavior and to psychic or psychotic manifestations" (Goldberg 1973). This problem is, of course, now a matter of international concern and is acknowledged as part of what has been called the "risk profile" of any psychotropic drug. This profile incorporates potential risks to public health, to public safety, and to the well-being of the dominant social order.

In sum, then, it is apparent that after twenty years psychotropic drugs are now firmly established in our therapeutic armamentarium, and have been instrumental in strengthening an important biological link between psychiatry and medicine, to their mutual benefit. It is clear, however, that a more rational basis for psychotropic drug use in clinical practice will have to supersede the various misuses that inevitably attend all empirical remedies. There are reasonable grounds for anticipating that such knowledge will be acquired within the next twenty years.

REFERENCES

Blackwell, B. (1973). Psychotropic drugs in use today: the role of diazepam in medical practice. *Journal of the American Medical Association* 225(13):1637.

Blackwell, B., and Marley, E. (1966). Interaction of cheese and its constituents with monoamine oxidase inhibitors. *British Journal of Pharmacology* 26:120.

Blackwell, B., and Shepherd, M. (1968). Prophylactic Librium: another therapeutic myth? *Lancet* 1:968.

Carlsson, A., Persson, T., Roos B.-E., and Walinder, J. (1972). Potentiation of phenothiazines by a-methyltyrosine in treatment of chronic schizophrenia. *Journal of Neural Transmission* 33, 83.

Godber, G. (1973). On the state of the public health (1972). *Health Trends* 5:65.

Goldberg, L. (1973). Summary. In *Psychic Dependence,* ed. L. Goldberg, and F. Hoffmeister, p. 224. Bayer Symposium IV. Berlin: Springer-Verlag.

Hirsch, S., Gaind, R., Rohde, P., Stevens, B., and Wing, J.K. (1973). Outpatient maintenance treatment of chronic schizophrenics with fluphenazine decanoate injection: a double blind placebo trial. *British Medical Journal* 1:633.

Keller, M. H., and McCurdy, R. L. (unpublished). Medical practice without anti-anxiety drugs.

Kimbell, L., Overall, J. E., and Hollister, L. E. (1965). Antidepressant drugs: myth or reality? *Journal of New Drugs* 5: 9.

Lewis, A. (1959). The impact of psychotropic drugs on the structure, function and future of psychiatric services. (a) In the hospitals. *Neuropsychopharmacology* 1:207.

Medical Research Council, Report by its Clinical Committee (1965). Clinical trial of the treatment of depressive illness. *British Medical Journal* 1:881.

Mindham, R. H. S., Howland, C., and Shepherd, M. (1973). An evaluation of continuation therapy with tricyclic antidepressants in depressive illness. *Psychological Medicine* 3:5.

Monitoring plasma concentrations of psychotropic drugs. (1974). *Drug and Therapeutics Bulletin* 12(2):6.

Ödegaard, Ö. (1964). Pattern of discharge from Norwegian psychiatric hospitals before and after the introduction of the psychotropic drugs. *American Journal of Psychiatry* 12:772.

Rashkis, H. A., and Smarr, E. R. (1958). A method for the control and evaluation of socio-psychological factors in pharmacological research. *Psychiatric Research Reports* (American Psychiatric Association) 9:21.

Sargant, W., and Slater, E. T. O. (1944). *An Introduction to Physical Methods of Treatment in Psychiatry.* Edinburgh: Livingstone.

Shepherd, M. (1961a). The influence of specific and nonspecific factors on the clinical effects of psychotropic drugs. In *Neuropsychopharmacology,* ed. E. Rothlin, p. 183. Amsterdam: Elsevier.

Shepherd, M. (1961b). The present status of psychopharmacology. *Journal of Chronic Diseases* 13:289.

Shepherd, M. (1964). The effectiveness of drugs in relationship to psychological and social forms of treatment. *Neuropsychopharmacology,* 3, ed. P.B. Bradley, F. Flugel, and P. Hoch, p. 139. Amsterdam, Elsevier, p. 139.

Shepherd, M., Lader, M., and Lader, S. (1968). Central nervous system depressant drugs. In *Side Effects of Drugs,* vol. 6, ed. I. Meyler and A. Herxheimer. Amsterdam: Excerpta Medica Foundation.

Shepherd, M., Lader, M., and Rodnight, R. (1968). *Clinical Psychopharmacology.* London: English University Press.

Shepherd, M., and Watt, D.C. (1975). Impact of long-term neuroleptics on the community: advantages and disadvantages. In *Neuropsychopharmacology,* ed. J.R. Boissier, H. Hippius, and P. Pichot, p. 379. Amsterdam and New York: Excerpta Medica.

Teeling-Smith, G. (1973). Psychotropic drugs and society. In: The medical use of psychotropic drugs. *Journal of the Royal College of General Practitioners.* Supplement No. 2:23, 58.

Weigert, E. (1973). The future of analysis. *Psychiatric News* 8:11.

World Health Organization Technical Report Series No. 371 (1967). *Research in Psychopharmacology.* Geneva: WHO.

Part I

Drugs

Chapter 2

The Classification of Psychotropic Drugs

The urge to classify knowledge has preoccupied Western thinking since the era of classical Greece. One of the most searching attempts to account for the fundamental importance of this activity was provided by William James, who suggested that, while the pure sciences expressed no more than the results of comparison, the truths of comparison were to be found in systems of classification. "It is, for some unknown reason, a great esthetic delight for the mind to break the order of experience," wrote James, "and class its materials in serial orders, proceeding from step to step of difference, and to contemplate, untiringly, the coursings and inosculations of the series among themselves. The first steps in most of the sciences are purely classificatory" (James 1950).

The growth of modern science has been accompanied by an increasing awareness of the need for a taxonomic thinking, the theoretical and practical value of which has been established in most fields of inquiry (Gregg 1954).

Practicing scientists as well as philosophers of science have come to accept the importance of classificatory systems, and James's conclusions have been echoed by Seymour Kety, one of the few eminent contemporary scientists with personal experiences of pharmacology and psychiatry: "Fundamentally, classification is an essential part of the process by which science comes to grips with the Universe," writes Kety. "It is essential in structuring the search for more information and in meaningfully and effectively communicating what has been learned: for these reasons it must occur very early in the scientific process" (Kety 1968).

HISTORY

The short history of modern psychopharmacology, a federation of disciplines still barely twenty years of age (Shepherd, Lader, and Rodnight 1968), illustrates the substance of Kety's view as well as the difficulties it poses. While some of these difficulties are specific to a complex and rapidly developing subject, many of them are rooted in the more general problems that confront the classification of all substances used in therapeutics. Some mention must, therefore, be made of the origin and nature of these difficulties if the varied and confusing attempts to classify psychotropic drugs are to be fully understood.

Perhaps the most influential early attempt to subdivide drugs in terms of their therapeutic effects was Cullen's *A Treatise of the Materia Medica* (1798). Cullen was much influenced by the Galenic system and arranged substances "according to their agreeing in some general virtues," in an attempt to match drugs with general therapeutic indications, thus helping the physician to choose compounds appropriate to the desired effect. The value of Cullen's modern-sounding approach was, however, limited by the paucity of pharmacologic knowledge in the eighteenth century, as becomes clear from his use of such categories as tonica, stimulantia, and astringentia.

With the advent of the scientific era in the nineteenth century and the many new chemicals then becoming available, the outlines of a fundamental difference in the approach to drug classification became apparent in the positions taken up by two major figures. For Claude Bernard, holding to his credo of experimental medicine, "toxic and medicinal action . . . come back to simple physiological changes in properties of the histological limits of our tissues"; thus "it is not enough for experimenting physicians to know that quinine cures fever; but what is above all significant to them is knowing what fever is and accounting for the mechanisms by which quinine cures" (Bernard 1957). In the field of drug action the logical consequences of this approach were to be developed by J. N. Langley and Paul Ehrlich, in the notion of chemoreceptors, which has since stirred many pharmacologists to try to construct "an ordering principle by which drug actions can be classified" (Schild 1968), in some manner possibly akin to the periodic table in organic chemistry.

The theoretical assumptions implicit in this view were contested by Rudolph Virchow (1959), who with his customary directness stated that—

> While I very gladly recognize the scientific seriousness of the effects of the physiological pharmacologist and wish him great success, I must, nevertheless, state in opposition that this cannot be the shortest path to the foundation of *reliable* therapy. . . . I would even prefer to leave it an open question whether this is the shortest path to the foundation of *rational* therapy. These attempts to pilot "rational" pathology and therapy under full sail—"rational" signifying

> that which reasonably explains the phenomena—resemble the attempts of Icarus. Why explanations, when what is to be explained is lacking? Let us first determine what it is that remedies do in diseases, and we shall soon learn how they do it.

Time has demonstrated the truth in both sides of the argument. Virchow's argument that a science of therapeutics would arise from a union between clinical experience and what he calls "pathological physiology," binding together "practical experiences in a gradually developing scientific order," tends to emphasize the therapeutic effects of a drug rather than its mode of action. The need to take more than one set of criteria into account, however, has been reflected in modern attempts to classify drugs. Sollmann (1957) puts the matter clearly:

> Systems of classifying drugs with systematic actions are unsatisfactory, because most drugs produce several effects which, by their interaction, complicate the subject so that no simple system will apply. With some drugs, one pharmacological, chemical or physical feature predominates so greatly that they can be separated as fairly distinct groups. . . . The pharmacological action in this sense is often not the therapeutic action. . . . For this reason it would not be advisable to classify drugs strictly according to their pharmacological actions. On the other hand, a *therapeutic classification* is not favorable to a study of the underlying actions of the drugs, and tends to empiricism.

From this argument it follows that drugs should be grouped "according to their principal pharmacological characters, taking account of all the important actions, as well as of the chemical properties, and in many cases also of the therapeutic uses of the drugs."

TRADITIONAL SUBDIVISIONS

Where the major biological action of a class of compounds overlaps in large measure its therapeutic effects, a single category can satisfy the pharmacologist and the clinician: the antibiotics may be taken as representative of such a drug class. However, the majority of drug categories contain a heterogeneous group of compounds, and none is less satisfactory than the rag-bag of drugs grouped together by virtue of their action on the central nervous system. The traditional subdivision into stimulants and depressants, along with a mixture of anticonvulsants, has entailed the inclusion of an unusually variegated group of compounds whose uneasy cohabitation has been strained still further by the arrival of a host of new drugs with psychotropic effects. Thus the British National Formulary, drawn up by a joint committee representing the medical and phamaceutical professions, and designed to "serve the usual requirements of most prescribers, whether in hospital or general practice," includes the following categories of drugs acting on the nervous system: analgesics, hypnotics, sedatives and tranquilizers, antidepressants, anticonvulsants, anti-Parkinsonian agents, cholinergic drugs, neuromuscular blocking drugs, and local anesthetics (British National Formulary 1968).

The current situation is not helped by the discordant definition of such terms as *sedation, hypnosis,* and *tranquilization.* On the one hand, for example, the British National Formulary includes sedatives with tranquilizers as drugs "intended to diminish certain unpleasant feelings without impairing alertness, a differential effect which no drug completely achieves. The feelings are those of tension, worry, anxiety, restlessness and panic." According to the Monthly Index of Medical Specialties (MIMS) classification, on the other hand, "The distinction between sedatives and hypnotics is mainly a question of dosage. Small doses of hypnotic produce sedation . . . the main difference between the tranquilizers and the traditional sedatives seems to depend on the fact that while large (hypnotic) doses of a sedative produce deep sleep and coma, little or no drowsiness occurs after large doses of a tranquilizer" (Pullom 1970). Again, the British Department of Health and Social Security subdivides psychotropic drugs into five groups—barbiturate hypnotics, nonbarbiturate hypnotics, tranquilizers, stimulants and appetite suppressants, and antidepressants—and so creates yet another set of criteria (Department of Health and Social Security 1969).

The Council on Drugs of the American Medical Association has recommended that psychotropic drugs be allocated, whenever possible, to existing categories on the basis of their human pharmacology (American Medical Association 1960), but a glance at some standard textbooks serves to illustrate the difficulties standing in the way of such a procedure. The ninth edition of Clark's *Applied Pharmacology,* for example, which has been described as "a textbook of therapeutics from the point of view of a pharmacologist" (Gaddum 1960), contains nine chapters under the general heading "Pharmacology of the Central Nervous System"; these cover such topics as the anesthetics, the hypnotics, alcohol, the analeptics, the central depressants of motor function, and the analgesics. A separate chapter on "Drugs Affecting Mental Activity" includes lysergic acid diethylamide, mescaline, chlorpromazine, reserpine, meprobamate, benactyzine, the amphetamines, methylphenidate, caffeine, and cocaine—along with electroconvulsive therapy (Wilson and Schild 1959). Laurence's *Clinical Pharmacology* brings together tranquilizers, antidepressants, and psychotomimetics in a chapter entitled "Drugs in Mental Disorder, Psychotomimetics" (Laurence 1966). Goodman and

Gilman (1965) employ an even more uncompromisingly therapeutic approach by including "Drugs Used in the Treatment of Psychiatric Disorders" under "Drugs Acting on the Central Nervous System" and subdividing them into "Drugs and Psychoses," "Drugs for Anxiety," "Drugs for Depression," and "Psychotogenic Drugs." By contrast, the text by Paton and Payne, claiming to "arrange its material according to bodily functions rather than drug groups" (Paton and Payne 1968), allocates antidepressants to a chapter on the control of consciousness, tranquilizers to the chapter on control of pain.

ATTEMPTS AT CLASSIFICATION OF PSYCHOTROPIC DRUGS

Against this background it is nonetheless instructive to examine the efforts of workers with a specialized interest in the field to classify psychotropic drugs. Following the early studies by Wundt, Kraepelin, and their colleagues in "pharmacopsychology," a remarkable attempt to do justice to the complexity of the situation was made by Louis Lewin in respect of "agents capable of effecting a modification of the cerebral functions, and used to obtain at will agreeable sensations of excitement or peace of mind" (Lewin 1931). Lewin's suggested categories were (1) euphoriants, the "sedatives of mental activity"; (2) phantastica, or "hallucinating substances"; (3) inebriantia, inducing "a primary phase of cerebral excitation . . . followed by a state of depression which may eventually extend to complete temporary suppression of the functions"; (4) hypnotica, or "sleep producing agents"; and (5) excitantia, "mental stimulants . . . which produce without alteration of consciousness a generally more or less apparent excitation of the brain." Despite their originality and clinical relevance, however, Lewin's views appear to have exercised little influence on the mainstream of pharmacological opinion.

The introduction of the phenothiazines, the Rauwolfia compounds, and meprobamate in the early 1950s ushered in an era of new psychotropic compounds and reawakened an interest in classification. Clinicians at first attempted to classify these compounds by employing a variety of colorful terms, such as *tranquilizers, ataractics, neuroleptics,* and *deturmoilizers,* even though it was even then pointed out that such words "define nothing and produce considerable confusion" (Irwin 1959). Several detailed schemata for clinical application were also proposed, and one of these, emanating from Delay and his co-workers in Paris, has been influential enough to demand consideration.

According to the French system, three large classes of drugs should be recognized by virtue of their action on mental activity, expressed in terms of *abatement, elevation,* or *deviation* (Delay 1959). The first class of compound is called the *psycholeptics,* a term which replaces the sedatives as a "group of medications that provide a decline in mental tonus, whether their principal action lies in the reduction of intellectual activity, or in the decrease of alertness, or in the sedation of emotional tension." The psycholeptics are subdivided into (1) the hypnotics, characterized by their predominant action on the function of sleep—for example, barbiturates; (2) the tranquilizers, which include meprobomate and benactyzine; and (3) the neuroleptics which contain chlorpromazine and the butyrophenones. It is postulated that the functional distinction between these subgroups is that the barbiturates, "being typical of the hypnotic drugs, are only simple sedatives or tranquilizers, when taken in small doses"; the tranquilizers are "characterized by their sedative action on anxiety and, to a certain degree, on agitation. They are sedatives in the classical sense of the word." By contrast, the neuroleptics are characterized by "a remarkable reductive action on psychotic processes" and by "a neurological syndrome composed of several elements: neurovegetative modification, psychomotor inhibition, disturbance of tonus, and occasionally abnormal motions of the extrapyramidal type."

The second class of compounds, the *psychoanaleptics*, are defined as drugs "capable of provoking an elevation of mental tonus," though their action "may lie in the enhancement of intellectual activity, or increase of alertness or uplift of mental tonus." Originally they included the amphetamines, methylphenidate, and isoniazid, and now contain a large group of compounds developed for the treatment of depressive illnesses.

For the third class of compounds the term *psychodysleptics* was introduced to indicate the "characteristic action of deviating mental activity and distorting appreciation of reality values." These drugs include such compounds as mescaline, lysergic acid diethylamide, and psilocybin.

An outline of this three-class schema is provided in Table 2-1. It has been widely publicized and, with some modifications, forms the basis of the provisional classification recommended by a special committee of the World Health Organization (1967) (Table 2-2). It deserves attention, however, less for its possible merits than for the general issues raised by its several deficiencies.

In the first place, the use of a new terminology barely disguises the grouping of psychotropic drugs into three global categories—sedating, stimulating, and psychotomimetic—a procedure crude enough to have been compared with that of "the classical anatomist who, with his scalpel, differentiated between muscle and bone" (Heimann 1969). Second, it illustrates well the tendency of so-called psychiatric anthropocentrism (Irwin 1968), a process whereby drugs are classified by a supposedly main or principal action in terms of a putative therapeutic effect, with scant regard to pharmacological or other

Table 2-1
Delay's Classification of Psychotropic Drugs

	Examples
A. Psycholeptics:	
acting on mental tonus ('nooleptics')	
1. *Hypnotics*	Barbiturates Non-barbiturate hypnotics
acting on mood ('thymoleptics')	
2. *Neuroleptics*	Phenothiazines Reserpine and its congeners Butyrophenones
3. *Tranquillizers*	Procalmadiol Methamine-diazepoxide
B. Psychoanaleptics:	
1. *Stimulants of mental tonus* ('nooanaleptics')	Amphetamines and their derivatives
2. *Mood-stimulants* ('thymoanaleptics'): Antidepressives	Diazepines Monoamine oxidase inhibitors
C. Psychodysleptics:	
Hallucinogenic or oneirogenic substances	Mescaline Lysergic acid diethyl-amide Psilocybin

Translated from Deniker (1966).

biological factors. Furthermore, the selection of one of many possible clinical actions of a drug is arbitrary and can be confusing—for example, the psycholeptics, selected as they are for their emphasis on sedation, are unlikely to include such nominally psychotomimetic compounds as ololiuqui or ibolaline, both of which can nonetheless induce markedly sedative effects; again, among psychoanaleptics, some of the tricyclic compounds can exert a sedative effect on normal subjects, while amphetamine can occasionally induce an atypically sedative rather than excitatory action.

Within the first two broad categories of the French schema the subcategories (see Table 2-1) raise problems of their own (Lambert and Revel 1969). In one major respect, as Kline (1969) has pointed out, the system is internally illogical:

> Delay and Deniker in their original publication referred to chlorpromazine as a "neuroleptic" because it produced extrapyramidal symptoms. The rest of the universe classifies chlorpromazine and other phenothiazines and phenothiazine-like drugs by the antipsychotic effect they have on the psychological state of the user. . . . Why the system should be disrupted by the inclusion of one category based on neurological side-effects is difficult to comprehend.

While accepting the justice of this comment, we may also observe that within his own similar system of classification—with psychoinhibitors, psychoactivators, psychotomimetics, and combinations as main categories—Kline does little more than substitute the term *ataraxis* for

Table 2-2
Classification of Psychotropic Drugs Recommended by Special Committee of WHO

Category	*Representative members*
Neuroleptics	*a.* Phenothiazines *b.* Butyrophenones *c.* Thioxanthenes *d.* Reserpine derivatives, benzoquinolizines
Anxiolytic sedatives	*a.* Meprobamate and derivatives *b.* Diazepoxides *c.* Barbiturates
Antidepressants	*a.* Monoamine oxidase (MAO) inhibitors *b.* Imipramine and other tricyclic compounds
Psychostimulants	*a.* Amphetamine, methylphenidate, pipradrol *b.* Caffeine
Psychodysleptics (hallucinogens)	*a.* Lysergic acid diethylamide (LSD) *b.* Mescaline *c.* Psilocybin *d.* Dimethyltryptophan (DMT) *e.* Cannabis (marihuana, hashish, etc.)

World Health Organization (1967).

neuroleptics to cover drugs which "remove, reverse, restrict or inhibit psychopathology, including hallucinations and delusions" (Freyhan 1961). By so doing he incorporates the controversial notion of *antipsychotic action,* a term which has proved notoriously difficult to define. According to Pöldinger (1965), for example,

> The designation "antipsychotic" does not mean the causal action on psychotic states: however, the term is supposed to describe an action which is more than the total of its partial effects on individual symptoms. The expression "more than the total" is reminiscent of the so-called "Gestaltpsychologie."

In the treatment of the schizophrenias this gestalt view of drug-action has been supported by some reports. Thus, the United States Psychopharmacology Service Center Collaborative Study Group (1964) conclude on the basis of their findings:

> Almost all symptoms and manifestations characteristic of schizophrenic psychoses improved with drug therapy, suggesting that the phenothiazines should be regarded as "antischizophrenic" in the broad sense. In fact, it is questionable whether the term "tranquilizer" should be retained.

Against this view, however, there is the clinical opinion of the many workers who attribute the therapeutic action of such compounds as the phenothiazines to their symptomatic effect on overactive behavior and who aver that such drug action can be seen as antischizophrenic only if the symptomatology of schizophrenia be equated with the disease process. In the present state of knowledge this must be regarded as a wholly unwarranted assumption: it has been shown, for example, that the degree of withdrawal in some schizophrenics can be related to the overactivity of some central nervous system functions (Venables and Wing 1962).

TARGET SYMPTOMS

A more widespread flirtation with the concept of specific drug action has been made by some workers with respect to individual psychopathological phenomena. It is implicit in Kline's subdivision of psychoactivators into "psychomotor stimulants," "psychostimulants," and "psychic energizers," and in Pöldinger's statement that "global action against depression can be divided into the following partial effects (Kielholz): mood-lifting of thymoleptic action (Schmidlin); unblocking of inhibition or thymeretic action (Janzarik); sedation of anxiety and agitation or neuroleptic action (Delay)" (Pöldinger 1965). Underlying this approach is the cloudy notion of the target symptom, advanced "in order to identify, if possible, those dysfunctions manifested by clinical symptoms which prove drug-treatable" (Freyhan 1965). This view cannot be sustained against two major objections. First, there is the difficulty of establishing reliable criteria of agreement on psychiatric symptomatology in view of the marked inter-observer variation which contributes so much to the difficulties of clinical assessment in psychiatry (Shepherd, Brooke, Cooper, and Lin 1968). Second, the traditional psychiatric symptoms enter into so many diagnostic categories that there is a wide range of conditions for which identical psychotropic drugs are prescribed. This point is largely conceded by Freyhan (1965), a principal advocate of the target symptom, when he admits that he "never intended to treat target symptoms as isolated phenomena in a nosological vacuum. Psychopathological states represent more than a sum total of separate symptoms." He goes on to enter a plea for "the 'double book-keeping system,' which envisages symptoms as integral components of psychopathological states. Accordingly, the therapeutic effects, momentary or substantial, depend on the relevant pathogenetic factors associated with schizophrenic, affective and brain disorders."

A further indication of the pitfalls attending the use of target symptomatology in this way is provided by the evidence that not only may different phenomena respond to the same drug but also that "psychopathological phenomena, often referred to as 'target symptoms,' labeled identically in different patients, respond differently to the same medication" (Klein and Davis 1969). In consequence, some research workers have gone so far as to discard diagnostic categories based on both the traditional rubrics and clinical symptomatology in favor of a "descriptive behavioral typology" worked out in terms of clinicostatistical analysis. Drug response, according to one biometric opinion, "appears to cut across traditional diagnostic groupings and yields a new basis for classifying psychiatric patients" (Clyde 1968). Attempts to apply this approach, however, have encountered difficulties of their own, as illustrated by the following:

> when the trait of "panic" is associated with auditory hallucinations, it should be weighted positively for beneficial chlorpromazine effect. However, in the presence of agoraphobia it should be weighted negatively. The implication is that "panic^1" is simply not the same as "panic^2" and identical coding of these two phenomenally similar behaviors does violence to the possibility of determining their relationships correctly. Formulating such complexities requires interaction terms that are not part of the usual additive multivariate approach. Furthermore, these interaction terms are very difficult if not impossible to establish on a statistical inductive basis. They may require stipulation

> derived from clinical experience. In turn, this would require a new level of creative interaction between clinicians and statisticians.
>
> Once patterned clinical diagnoses were developed it would still be necessary to show that the application of these patterns led to predictions of drug effects on specific aspects of the pattern that would be significantly better than predictions that utilized data in univariate fashion or in the form of linear additive multiple regression equations. In any case, the issue of diagnosis has not been avoided by the attempts to relate symptom reduction directly to drug effects, but rather has been reemphasized as an investigative area. [Klein 1968]

CLINICOPATHOLOGICAL CRITERIA

Some clinicians have acknowledged the intrinsic difficulties of a purely clinical classification of psychotropic drugs by incorporating other criteria into their systems. Lehmann, for example, has elaborated a triple subdivision into drugs which induce inhibition, excitation, and psychotomimesis respectively, by distinguishing three types of therapeutic action which might be applied to the drug treatment of psychiatric patients: (1) a "curative" action, when the cause is known and can be eliminated—for example, penicillin for GPI; (2) a "corrective" action, when an agent can influence a whole pattern of functions or a syndrome that characterizes a particular illness—for example, insulin for diabetes, digitalis for heart disease, and tranquilizing drugs in "a number of acute and chronic psychotic conditions"; and (3) a "symptomatic" action, when therapy is aimed at particular symptoms such as pain or insomnia, which may be unrelated to etiology but "rather remote and indirect manifestations of secondary functional deviations within the general picture of the disease." Examples of such symptomatic action might be morphine for pain, barbiturates for insomnia, and chlorpromazine for the immediate reduction of severe psychomotor excitement (Lehmann 1959). In addition, Lehmann advances a hypothetical rationale for drug action, not only by postulating three functional systems in the central nervous apparatus—a visceropsychic system, a sensoripsychic system, and a corticopsychic system (Lehmann 1956)—but by proposing arousal, affect, and integration as three "comprehensive parameters of human psychic functioning," each with "an anatomical representation in specific units of the central nervous system," as a basis for classification (Lehmann 1963).

It should be emphasized, however, that there is very little empirical support for such views. Their interest resides more in the objective to which they aspire, a goal Freyhan has defined as "the foundations of a new classification which integrates basic structural models of chemical components with basic effect patterns on clinical syndromes " (Freyhan 1965). He continues: "It may not be too farfetched to anticipate chemical approaches to experimental psychopathology which will utilize the response affinity of syndromes to specific chemical constituents as the basis for decoding the still mysterious network of pathogenic links and factors." Whether or not this goal is farfetched, it must remain remote as long as such chemically similar compounds as imipramine, carbamazepine, and chlorpromazine can exert such unpredictably dissimilar clinical actions.

This yearning by clinicians for a pathophysiological basis to underpin a clinical classification of psychiatric disease is matched by an awareness on the part of some neuropharmacologists of the need to include clinical criteria within an essentially biological schema. The difficulties created by a disregard for clinical phenomena are linked to an understandable desire to simplify the field of enquiry by restricting experimental data to animal responses and then assuming that human and animal responses are coterminous. The merits and limitations of this assumption have been pointed out by Cook (1965)

> It has been shown that when man is studied under experimental conditions similar to those used with animals, the measured behavior is similar to that seen in animals and the drug effects are similar. This certainly adds support to the generality of the measured behavior and drug effects and the usefulness of such animal studies as functional analogues of human behavior. However, in addressing ourselves to the relationship of such studies to the clinical syndrome, we find that the question of relevance of the similar drug effects in animals and man to the therapeutic action in the clinical syndrome is yet to be determined.

Imipramine furnishes an excellent illustration for Cook's comment. Writing of Kuhn's clinical acumen in observing the clinical effects of this derivative with marked structural and pharmacological similarities to the phenothiazines, Klerman and Cole (1965) emphasize that "the available data gave no indication of the possible antidepressant effects of imipramine. On the contrary, all the indications were that it was similar to chlorpromazine." It was, in fact, the clinical action of imipramine which led to the search for biological effects distinguishing it from the phenothiazines and to which, in the opinion of many workers, its antidepressant action must be attributed.

BIOLOGICAL CLASSIFICATIONS

Despite the preceding considerations, attempts to furnish a strictly biological classification of psychotropic drugs have not been lacking, with animal workers favoring chemical or pharmacological criteria (Giurgea 1969

Janssen 1970) and clinical investigators tending toward electrophysiological responses (Fink 1968). The neurobiologists' case against such endeavors has been summarized by Toman (1962):

> Most classifications for didactic purposes are hybrid, traditional, colorful, and misleading. The chief reason for this unsatisfactory state of affairs is the relative poverty of knowledge concerning mechanisms, either at the cellular or molecular levels of explanation, which would give a sound theoretical base for systematizing drugs.

The most clearheaded recognition of this comment, and of the conceptual problems involved in any biological classification of psychotropic drugs, is contained in the schema of Jacobsen (1963), who has argued that at present "we have no better method of classifying psychotropic drugs than to place compounds with similar effects together, irrespective of their chemical constitutions." On the basis of data from animal experiments which provide information about drug effects on different levels and functions of the central nervous system, Jacobsen (1959) has pointed out that only a "profile of action" of a drug can do comprehensive justice to the experimental results obtained: otherwise the categorization of the same compound will vary with the particular axis of classification that is selected. He concludes: "If attempts must be made to place chemically and pharmacologically related compounds in strict relation to each other, then a multidimensional system is necessary" (1958). However, Jacobsen also recognizes the importance of the interrelation between pharmacodynamic and clinical effects, requiring of a fully multidimensional biological classification system the inclusion of several categories derived from drug action on patients and normal subjects.

OBSTACLES TO A SATISFACTORY CLASSIFICATION

In sum, the obstacles to satisfactory classification in psychopharmacology reside partly in our ignorance about psychotropic drugs and partly in that about mental illness. With regard to the former, Elkes (1967) has justly commented:

> The inordinately wide range of action of the psychotropic drugs introduced special difficulties. As is well known, their influence on thought-process behavior is but one of their effects. Most (indeed all) have a widespread range of action on physiological targets outside the CNS, making their psychotropic features special instances of more general phenomena. The question of precise and relevant criteria to serve as a basis for a classification therefore forces itself on the subject from the outset; and here, as elsewhere, the lack of positive guidelines only emphasizes the lack of definition of the field as a whole.

Against the background of these difficulties, Elkes concludes that no satisfactory classification can be based on chemical effects, pharmacological effects on peripheral drug receptors, psychophysiological central effects, or effects on animal behavior; further, the subjective and objective drug effects in man constitute a field which can be so confusing as to demand a "carefully calibrated glossary" from the outset.

With regard to the conditions for which the various psychopharmacologic compounds are prescribed in clinical practice, it is apparent that if the status of classification within a branch of medicine is taken as an index of established knowledge, then psychiatry is a poorly developed specialty. The reasons for this have been succinctly summarized by Zubin (1968):

> Disease is usually defined in terms of "etiology," "structure," and "symptomatology." In most mental disorders

> etiology is unknown, the structure of the organs of the patients . . . unaffected, and symptomatology is the only available basis for the definition.

After more than fifty years, Bleuler's comment on the various forms of schizophrenia, that it is "not a question of defining diseases but of grouping symptoms," remains true not only of the schizophrenias but also of the great majority of all mental disorders. Another equally important factor is that the Linnaean basis of biological subdivision applies less to mental illness than to physical disease, so as to justify Lewis's verdict that "the problems and purposes of psychiatric classification are more akin to those of the ecologist than of the morphologist" (Lewis 1952). Accordingly, any form of classification which depends on therapeutic response must be suspect.

WHAT SHOULD BE DONE?

What, then, can be done at the present time? The increasing volume of knowledge about the manifold aspects of psychotropic drugs and the rapidly changing stage of this knowledge highlight the need for a comprehensive classification of psychotropic drugs. The preparation of such a classification would be a complex task, especially as the classification would have to be capable of accommodating many changes. In addition, the formation by the World Health Organization of International Reference Centers for psychopharmacology makes it clear that some form of universally acceptable classification is becoming urgently necessary (Leeds 1970).

A psychotropic drug classification might emerge from the application of what information scientists call "facet analysis," a procedure which first groups the terms into categories—kind, state, property, reaction, operation, device, and so on—and then arranges the terms within each category into the form of a classificatory map (Vickery 1959). The application of this technique could be an integral part of the systematic collection of information about psychotropic drugs (see Appendix). The value of such an approach in the sphere of information retrieval has already been demonstrated in other branches of medicine (McClelland and Mapleson 1966, Barkla 1969). Considerable experience of the mechanization of some of the processes, which are essential components of information services, has been accumulated (Pickford 1968, 1969). By the use of a faceted, precoordinate, open-ended system for indexing the basic data relating to psychotropic drugs, a flexible classification could emerge from the information system. This approach of allowing a classification to be developed from the experience of a working information service is thought preferable to the imposition of a preconceived schema. A specialized information center, with the task of developing a classification on the lines indicated, could be usefully set up in the near future.

APPENDIX

HELEN MARSHALL, M.A., A.L.A.
Librarian, Institute of Psychiatry

When a paper is indexed for future retrieval, a precoordinate or postcoordinate system may be used. In the former the headings given to the paper are related, or coordinated, at the time of indexing—that is, before the entry is filed. In a postcoordinate system, on the other hand, each heading is dealt with separately and it is only later, when the paper is being retrieved, that two or more headings are linked. In a precoordinate system a classification scheme may be used to arrange the headings in a particular order: if the scheme is a faceted one, the subject matter of the paper is analyzed according to the different facets covered and these facets can then be regrouped in any desired combination or combinations. In either system a controlled vocabulary, or thesaurus, is compiled to cover the terms customarily found in the literature and to show under which preferred heading such terms should be indexed. If a classification scheme is used, the thesaurus will also show where in the scheme a given preferred heading comes.

A paper dealing with suicide in patients receiving antidepressant drugs might, for example, be indexed under suicide, depression, and antidepressant drugs—let us say headings, A, B and C. In a postcoordinate system, three entries only would be made, under A, B, and C. In a faceted precoordinate system the symbols would be rotated to give the permutation ABC, BAC, BCA, CAB, ACB, and six entries would go into the file, in classified order: this number could, if desired, be reduced by rotating selectively instead of permuting. At the point of retrieval, in most postcoordinate systems the searcher would select the three headings A, B, and C, and would look at each separately, to discover which entry numbers were common to all three. In a precoordinate system a searcher interested in suicide generally could find all suicide entries together—suicide, general (A), suicide in depressed patients (AB), and suicide in depressed patients receiving drugs (ABC). The precoordinate system thus gives a broader, more organized view of suicide, but at the expense of having a larger number of entries. If papers receive, on the average, three headings each, the number of permuted entries should be manageable; if papers are indexed in depth, however, with perhaps up to ten entries each, the problems raised by permutation may be considerable. It is perhaps relevant to mention here that in the printed Index Medicus each entry appears, on the average, under three headings, although up to 10 may be entered against it on the associated computer tape.

Since psychopharmacology is a wide-ranging subject, and since it is not easy to obtain an overall view of its different aspects, it would seem reasonable to try first the precoordinate faceted approach mentioned in Professor Shepherd's last paragraph. An attempt has therefore been made to index a small number of titles in a small section of the field and to coordinate and permute the different facets that emerged. The material consisted of the forty-two titles listed in Appendix Table 2-1, covering papers on dibenzazepine compounds (or the tricyclic antidepressants, as they are more commonly called). Forty titles came from the cumulated volume of Psychopharmacology Abstracts for 1969 and two more were added to illustrate further aspects of the literature on anti-depressant drugs. No attempt was made to locate and read the papers, and abstracts were looked at only in two cases, to clear up doubts about the subject mattter.

The titles were indexed broadly according to the aspects of psychopharmacology with which they were concerned. A provisional code, or set of symbols, was added and these symbols were permuted to show all possible combinations (although in some cases selective rotation might have been enough). The titles were not indexed specifically or in depth, each receiving only two or three symbols to indicate their broad approach. From the titles used, the following main facets emerged: chemistry, pharmacology, psychology, sociology, diseases and their treatment, and adverse effects. Most of these were subdivided, again very broadly, and the resulting divisions are shown in Appendix Table 2-2.

Appendix Table 2-1
Titles of 42 papers on Tricyclic Antidepressants*

Title no.		*Provisional code*
1	Over-dosage of psychotropic drugs: II. Antidepressants	ST/PR
2	Nortriptyline hydrochloride in treatment of enuresis in mentally retarded boys	ST/MU/MHD
3	Behavioural facilitation: the interaction of imipramine and desipramine with amphetamine, alpha-pipradrol, methylphenidate and thozalinine	ST/IK
4	Drugs and dreams: III. The effects of imipramine on the dreams of depressed patients	ST/MR/IL
5	On the pharmacology of antidepressants of tricyclic structure	ST/F
6	The influence of several tricyclic compounds on the activity of monoamine oxidase of rat liver, brain and heart	ST/FF/FDE
7	A possible relationship between catecholamines and acute toxicity of desipramine	ST/FG/FDG
8	A double-blind trial of amitriptyl/perphenazine	ST/MR
9	Does the simultaneous administration of imipramine increase the efficacy of electric shock?	ST/MR
10	Sequential double-blind controlled trial of opipranol in anxiety neurosis	ST/MR
11	Pharmacotherapy of the depressions with protriptyline	ST/MR
12	Evaluation of the therapeutic action of nortriptyline in depressive syndromes	ST/MR
13	Comparative trial of nortriptyline and amitriptyline in 100 depressed patients	ST/MR
14	A double-blind evaluation of chlorprozamine v. a combination of perphenazine and amtriptyline	ST/MR
15	Intrahepatic obstructive jaundice from amitriptyline	ST/PH
16	Tofranil poisoning	ST/PH
17	Pharmacological sleep studies in man: pentobarbital, amitriptyline, chlordiazepoxide and RD.6901	ST/FDF
18	Metabolism of C-imipramine: I. Excretion in the rat and in man	ST/FF
19	The adrenal response to metyrapone in amitriptyline-treated subjects	ST/FE
20	Effects of imipramine on individuals in levels of depression	ST/IM
21	Tricyclic antidepressants (leading article)	ST
22	A double-blind trial of amitriptyl/perphenazine	ST/MR

*40 titles from *Psychopharmacology Abstracts* 9 (1969), plus 2 additional ones.

Appendix Table 2-1 (continued)
Titles of 42 papers on Tricyclic Antidepressants

Title no.		***Provisional code***
23	Medical and psychosocial factors in enuretic children treated with imipramine	ST/MHD/JH
24	Imipramine and amtriptyline treatment of enuresis in retarded children	ST/MU/MHD
25	Treating psychological disturbances induced by physical disorders: a double-blind study of perphenazine and amitriptyline in anxiety and depression	ST/MP/MH
26	Imipramine: effects on the dreams of the depressed	ST/MR/IL
27	The effect of desipramine injected intercerebrally in normal or reserpenized rats	ST/FDG
28	Position of nortriptyline in the group of antidepressive drugs, with clinical and EEG considerations	ST/MR/FDH
29	The relation role of storage and synthesis of brain norepinephrine in the psychomotor stimulation evoked by amphetamine or by desipramine and tetrabenazine	ST/FF/FDG
30	Desipramine in shizophrenic states	ST/MT
31	Systematic studies with trimipramine, a new antidepressant drug	ST/MR
32	The chemical structure of tricyclic antidepressants	ST/B
33	Comparative pharmacological characteristics of amitriptyline and imipramine	ST/F
34	A more effective method for the use of imipramine in depression	ST/MR
35	Myocardial damage in amitriptyline and nortriptyline poisoning	ST/PH
36	Demethylation of 12 tricyclic psychotropic drugs using rat liver microsomes	ST/FC
37	Protriptyline: a double-blind clinical trial	ST/MR
38	Desipramine, a thymoanaleptic with the major effect of motor inhibition	ST/FDF
39	Research on cardiac effects of nortriptyline: I. Study of response of isolated heart perfused with adrenaline and noradrenaline	ST/FDE
40	The therapeutic value of nortriptyline hydrochloride in severe depressive syndromes	ST/MR
41	The direct comparison of anti-depressants, imipramine and chlorprothixene	ST/MR
42	Problems posed by severe amitriptyline intoxications	ST/PH

Appendix Table 2-2

Provional Coding Derived From 42 Titles

B CHEMISTRY

F PHARMACOLOGY
- FC Biochemical, cellular, molecular, biophysical, drug mechanisms
- FD Physiological
  - FDE Systematic
    - FDF Central nervous system
      - FDG Brain
      - FDH Electroencephalography

I PSYCHOLOGY
- IK Behaviour
- IL Dreams
- IM Affect

J SOCIOLOGY
- JH Medical

M DISEASES
- MH Physical
  - MHD Enuresis
- MP Psychiatric
  - MR Depression
  - MT Schizophrenia
  - MU Mental retardation

P ADVERSE EFFECTS
- PH Physical
- PR Suicide, attempted suicide

S DRUGS
- ST Tricyclic antidepressants

The main facets coincide approximately, and not surprisingly, with corresponding "main-topic categories" used in the Classified Abstract Archive of the Alcohol Literature, although this was not taken as a guide. The subdivisions in pharmacology were chosen to follow the broad headings used by the *British Journal of Pharmacology.* The categories shown are not meant to be comprehensive: other main facets would have emerged if more titles had been used, and numerous subdivision would also be required.

Appendix Table 2-3 shows the forty-two titles arranged in classified order—that is, with each title appearing once only, in its place in the scheme. The titles have been arranged in a strict citation order, as if the tricyclic antidepressants were always the main topic of the paper,

Appendix Table 2-3

Titles Arranged in Classified Order

Code		Title number
ST	TRICYCLIC ANTIDEPRESSANTS	
	General	21
ST/B	Chemistry	32
ST/F	Pharmacology	5, 33
FC	biochemical, etc.	36
FDE	physiological	
	systematic	39
FDF	central nervous system	17, 38
FDG	brain	27
FE	autopharmacology	19
FF	pharmacokinetics	18
FF/FDE	—systematic	6
FDG	—brain	29
FG	toxicity	
FG/FDG	—brain	7
ST/I	Psychology	
IK	behaviour	3
IM	affect	20
ST/M	Diseases	
MHD/JH	enuresis—medical sociology	23
MP/MH	psychiatric—physical	25
MR	depression	8, 9, 10, 11, 12, 13, 14, 22, 31, 34, 37, 40, 41
MR/FDH	—EEG	28
/IL	—dreams	4, 26
MT	schizophrenia	30
MU	mental retardation	
MU/MHD	—enuresis	2, 24
ST/P	Adverse reactions	
PH	physical	15, 16, 35, 42
PR	**suicide, attempted suicide**	1

although this was not necessarily the case. Appendix Table 2-4 shows the additional entries obtained by permuting the symbols attached to each title.

No attempt was made to indicate whether an article was, for example, a case report, or a comprehensive review; or whether it dealt with animal experiments, controlled clinical trials, or drugs used in combination. A code could be provided to cover such points, as well as others like age and geographical or ethnic distribution; symbols of this kind would be applicable to any relevant entry in the file.

It must be emphasized again that this represents only a very crude attempt to show how a faceted index might be begun. Its aim would be to facilitate retrieval of documents on psychopharmacology, in the first instance, and it would grow, not by fitting drugs into pre-selected categories, but by letting the index show, as it developed, the groups into which they fell. It is hoped that such an index would eventually contribute toward a regrouping of psychopharmacological agents that would be useful to clinicians, pharmacologists, biochemists, and members of other disciplines concerned. A byproduct might be a general classification of psychiatric literature, which could be used in other special aspects of the subject, or cover the field as a whole.

Appendix Table 2-4
Additional Entries Obtained by Rotating the Codes

Code		*Title number*
B	CHEMISTRY	
B/ST	Tricyclics	32
F	PHARMACOLOGY	
F/ST	General—tricyclics	5, 33
FC/ST	Biochemical—tricyclics	36
FD	Physiological	
FDE/FF/ST	systematic—pharmacokinetics—tricyclics	6
ST	—tricyclics	39
ST/FF	—pharmacokinetics	6
FDF/ST	central nervous system—tricyclics	17, 38

Appendix Table 2-4 (continued)
Additional Entries Obtained by Rotating the Codes

Code		*Title number*
FDG/FF/ST	brain—pharmacokinetics—tricyclics	29
FG/ST	—toxicity—tricyclics	7
ST	—tricyclics	27
ST/FF	—tricyclics—pharmacokinetics	29
ST/FG	—tricyclics—toxicity	7
FDH/MR/ST	EEG—depression—tricyclics	28
ST/MR	tricyclics—depression	28
FE/ST	Autopharmacology—tricyclics	19
FF/FD/ST	Pharmacokinetics—systematic physiology—tricyclics	6
FDG/ST	brain—tricyclics	29
ST	—tricyclics	18
ST/FD	—systematic physiology	6
FDG	—brain	29
FG/FDG/ST	Toxicity—brain—tricyclics	7
ST/FDG	tricyclics—brain	7
I	PSYCHOLOGY	
IK/ST	Behaviour—tricyclics	3
IL/MR/ST	Dreams—depression—tricyclics	4, 25
ST/MR	tricyclics—depression	4, 25
IM/ST	Affect —tricyclics	20
J	SOCIOLOGY	
JH/MHD/ST	Medical—enuresis—tricyclics	23
ST/MHD	tricyclics—enuresis	23
M	DISEASES	
MH/MP/ST	Physical—psychiatric—tricyclics	25
ST/MP	tricyclics—psychiatric	25
MHD/JH/ST	enuresis—medical sociology—tricyclics	23
ST	mental retardation—tricyclics	2, 24
ST/JH	tricyclics—medical sociology	23
ST/MU	mental retardation	2, 24
MP/ST/MH	Psychiatric—physical—tricyclics	25
ST/MH	tricyclics—physical	25
MR/FDH/ST	depression—EEG—tricyclics	28
IL/ST	dreams—tricyclics	4, 26
ST	tricyclics	8, 9, 10, 11, 12, 13, 14, 22, 31, 34, 37, 40, 41
ST/FDH	tricyclics—EEG	28
ST/IL	dreams	4, 26
MT/ST	schizophrenia	30
MU/MHD/ST	mental retardation—enuresis—tricyclics	2, 24
ST/MDH	tricyclics—enuresis	2, 24
P	ADVERSE EFFECTS	
PH/ST	Physical—tricyclics	15, 16, 35, 42
PR/ST	Suicide, attempted suicide—tricyclics	1
ST	TRICYCLIC ANTIDEPRESSANTS	
ST/F	Pharmacology	
FDE/FF	systematic physiology—pharmacokinetics	6
FDG/FF	brain—pharmacokinetics	29
FG	toxicity	7
FDH/MR	EEG—depression	28
ST/IL/MR	Psychology—dreams—depression	4, 26
ST/JH/MHD	Sociology—medical—enuresis	23
ST/MH/MP	Diseases—physical—psychiatric	25
MHD/MU	enuresis—mental retardation	2, 24

REFERENCES

American Medical Association (1966). *New and Nonofficial Drugs.* Philadelphia: Lippincott.

Barkla, J. K. (1969). The University of Sheffield biomedical information project. *The Information Scientist* 3:13-20.

Bernard, C. (1957). *An Introduction to the Study of Experimental Medicine.* Trans. H. C. Greene. New York: Dover.

British National Formulary (1968). London: British Medical Association and the Pharmaceutical Society of Great Britain, p. 68.

Brodie, B. B. and Shore, P. A. (1959). Mechanism of action of psychotropic drugs. In *Psychopharmacology Frontiers,* ed. N. S. Kline, pp. 413-419. Boston: Little, Brown.

Clyde, D. J. (1968). Patterns of reaction to drug treatments derived through multivariate procedures. In *The Role and Methodology of Classification in Psychiatry and Psychopathology,* ed. M.M. Katz, J.O. Cole, and W.E. Barton, pp. 483-492. Washington: United States Department of Health, Education and Welfare.

Cook, L. (1965). Behaviour changes with antipsychotic drugs in animals. In *Neuropsychopharmacology,* vol. 4, ed. D. Bente and P. B. Bradley, pp. 91-99. Amsterdam: Elsevier.

Cullen, W. (1798). *A Treatise of the Materia Medica.* Vol. 1. Edinburgh: Elliott.

Delay, J. (1959). Discussion of pharmacologic treatment of schizophrenics. In *Psychopharmacology Frontiers,* ed. N. S. Kline, p. 426. Boston: Little, Brown.

Deniker, P. (1966). *La Psychopharmacologie.* Paris: Presse Universitaires de France.

Department of Health and Social Security (1969). Annual Report for the Year 1968. London: H.M.S.O.

Elkes, J. (1967). Behavioral pharmacology in relation to psychiatry. In *Psychiatrie der Gegenwart,* ed. H. W. Gruhle, R. Jung, W. Mayer-Gross, and M. Muller Band 1/1, Teil a, pp. 929-1038. Berlin: Springer.

Fink, M. (1968). E.E.G. classification of psychoactive compounds in man: a review and theory of behavioural associations. In *Psychopharmacology: a Review of Progress: 1957-1967,* ed.

D. H. Efron, J. O. Cole, J. Levine and J. R. Wittenborn. Washington, D.C.: Public Health Service Publication No. 1836.

Freyhan, F.A. (1961). On classifying psychotropic pharmaca. *Comprehensive Psychiatry* 2:241.

Freyhan, F. A. (1965). Dynamics and significance of psychopharmacological intervention in psychiatry. In *Neuropsychopharmacology*, ed. D. Bente and P. B. Bradley, pp. 249-254. Amsterdam: Elsevier.

Gaddum, J. H. (1940). *Pharmacology*. London: Oxford University Press, p. xiii.

Giurgea, C. (1969). Pharmacological criteria for the classification of tranquillizers. In *The Present Status of Psychotropic Drugs*, ed. A. Cerletti and F. J. Bovet, pp. 154-167. Amsterdam: Excerpta Medica.

Goodman, L. S. and Gilman, A., ed. (1965). *The Pharmacological Basis of Therapeutics*, 3rd ed., New York: Macmillan, p. 159.

Gregg, J. R. (1954). *The Language of Taxonomy*. New York: Columbia University Press.

Heimann, H. (1969). Effects of psychotropic drugs on normal man. *Confinia Psychiatrica* 12:205-221.

Irwin, S. (1959). Discussion of pharmacologic treatment of schizophrenics. In *Psychopharmacology Frontiers*, ed. N. S. Kline, p. 425. Boston: Little, Brown.

Irwin, S. (1968). A rational framework for the development, evaluation and use of psychoactive drugs. *American Journal of Psychiatry* 124 Supplement 1-19.

Jacobsen, E. (1959). The comparative pharmacology of some psychotropic drugs. *Bulletin of the World Health Organization* 21:411-419.

Jacobsen, E. (1963). The classification of psychotropic drugs. *Journal of Neuropsychiatry* 4:241-246.

James, W. (1950). *The Principles of Psychology*. Vol. 2. New York: Dover, p. 646.

Janssen, P. A. J. (1970). Chemical and pharmacological classification of neuroleptics. In *The Neuroleptics*, ed. D. P. Bobon, P. A. J. Janssen, and J. Bobon, pp. 33-44. Basle: Karger.

Kety, S. S. (1969). Problems in psychiatric nosology from the viewpoint of the biological sciences. In *The Role and Methodol-*

ogy of Classification in Psychiatry and Psychopathology, ed. M. M. Katz, J. O. Cole, and W. E. Barton, pp. 190-193. Washington, D.C.: United States Department of Health, Education and Welfare, Public Health Service Publication No. 1584.

Klein, D. F. (1968). Diagnosis and pattern of reaction to drug treatment: clinically derived formulations. In *The Role and Methodology of Classification in Psychiatry and Psychopathology,* ed. M. M. Katz, J. O. Cole, and W. E. Barton, pp. 466-481. Washington, D.C.: United States Department of Health, Education and Welfare.

Klein, D. F. and Davis, J. M. (1969). *Diagnosis and Drug Treatment of Psychiatric Disorders.* Baltimore: Williams and Wilkins, p. 448.

Klerman, G. L. and Cole, J. O. (1965). Clinical pharmacology of imipramine and related antidepressant compounds. *Pharmacological Review* 17:101.

Kline, N. S. (1969). Nomenclature vs. nature. *International Journal of Psychiatry* 7:292.

Lambert, P. A. and Revol, L. (1969). Classification of neuroleptics. *Comprehensive Psychiatry* 10:50.

Laurence, D. R. (1966). *Clinical Pharmacology.* London: Churchill, p. 299.

Leeds, A. A. (1970). A. W.H.O. reference center network for information on psychotropic drugs. In *The Neuroleptics,* 2nd ed., ed. D. P. Bobon, P. A. J. Jansen, and J. Bobon, pp. 164-167. Basle: Karger.

Lehmann, H. E. (1956). A dynamic concept of the action of chlorpromazine at physiological and psychological levels. *Encephale* 45:1113.

Lehmann, H. E. (1959). Concepts, rationale and research. In *Psychopharmacology Frontiers,* ed. N. S. Kline, pp. 21-30. Boston: Little, Brown.

Lehmann, H. E. (1963). Problems of evaluation and classification in psychopharmacology. In *Psychopharmacological Methods,* ed. Z. Votava, M. Horvath, and O. Vinar, pp. 276-280. Prague: State Medical Publishing House.

Lewin, L. (1931). *Phantastica, Narcotic and Stimulating Drugs.* Translated from the 2nd German edition by P. H. A. Wirth. London: Kegan Paul.

Lewis, A. (1952). The classification of schizophrenia. In *Psychiatrie Clinique,* pp. 247-256. Premier Congres Mondiale de Psychiatrie, Paris, 1950. Paris: Hermann.

Lewis, J. J. (1964). The classification of tranquilizers. *Practitioner* 192:12-22.

McClelland, R. M. A. and Mapleson, W. W. (1966). Feature cards. A method of indexing anaesthetic literature. *Anaesthesia* 21:3-18.

National Institute of Mental Health, Psychopharmacology Service Center Collaborative Study Group (1964). Phenothiazine treatment in acute schizophrenia. *Archives of General Psychiatry* 10:246-261.

Paton, W. D. M. and Payne, J. P. (1968). *Pharmacological Principles and Practice.* London: Churchill.

Pickford, A. G. A. (1968). An objective method for the generation of an information retrieval language. *Information Scientist* 2:17-37.

Pickford, A. G. A. (1969). 80-column cards as feature cards. *Information Scientist* 3:69-79.

Poldinger, W. (1965). *Discussion in Neuropsychopharmacology.* vol. 4, ed. D. Bente and P. B. Bradley, pp. 267-268. Amsterdam: Elsevier.

Pullon, E. N., ed. (1970). MIMS. *Annual Compendium 1969,* p. 8. London: Haymarket Press.

Schild, H. O. (1968). A pharmacological approach to drug receptors. In *Importance of Fundamental Principles in Drug Evaluation,* ed. D. H. Tedeschi and R. E. Tedeschi, p. 257. New York: Raven Press.

Shepherd, M., Brooke, E. M., Cooper, J. E. and Lin, T. (1968). An experimental approach to psychiatric diagnosis. *Acta Psychiatrica Scandinavica* Supplement 201.

Shepherd, M., Lader, M. and Rodnight, R. (1968). *Clinical Psychopharmacology.* London: English Universities Press.

Sollmann, T. (1957). *A Manual of Pharmacology.* 8th ed. Philadelphia: Saunders, p. 43.

Tolman, J. E. P. (1962). Neurotropic drugs. In *Neurochemistry,* ed. K. A. C. Elliott, I. H. Page, and J. H. Quastel, pp. 728-765. Springfield, Ill.: Thomas.

Venables, P. H., and Wing, J. K. (1962). Level of arousal and the subclassification of schizophrenia. *Archives of General Psychiatry* 7:114-119.

Vickery, B. C. (1959). *Classification and Indexing in Science.* London: Butterworths, p. 12.

Virchow, R. (1959). Scientific method and therapeutic standpoints. In *Disease, Life and Man,* trans. L. J. Rather, p. 55. Stanford, Cal.: Stanford University Press.

Wilson, A. and Schild, H. O. (1959). *Applied Pharmacology (Clark).* London: Churchill, p. 261.

World Health Organisation (1967). *Research in Psychopharmacology.* Technical Reprint Services, 371. Geneva: World Health Organization.

Zubin, J. (1968). Discussion in *The Role and Methodology of Classifications in Psychiatry and Psychopathology.* Ed. M.M. Katz, J.O. Cole, and W.E. Barton, p. 24. Washington: U.S. Department of Health, Education and Welfare.

Chapter 3

Reserpine as a "Tranquilizer"

Reserpine is one of the two most prominent representatives of that group of substances which have come to be widely known as the *tranquilizing agents.* I shall try to review briefly what has been learned about this drug, to summarize our own experience with it, and to indicate some of the important deficiencies in our knowledge, specifically about reserpine but, by extension, about its congeners as well.

The history of reserpine is by now a familiar one. Although it was not isolated until 1952 from the climbing shrub, *Rauwolfia serpentina* (Benth.), the powdered whole root of this plant had been used medicinally in India and nearby countries for many centuries in the treatment of diverse ailments. Pharmacologically, reserpine is the most active of the several Rauwolfia alkaloids which have so far been extracted; chemically, it is closely related to yohimbane. The discovery that the single alkaloid reserpine could be substituted for Rauwolfia in the treatment of hypertension stimulated interest in the numerous effects this drug produced; in addition to its hypotensive action, well-established observations show its effects to include miosis, bradycardia, increased motor and secretory gastrointestinal activity, lacrimation, respiratory inhibition, relaxation of the nictitating membrane, and hypothermia. Investigation of these effects by the classical techniques of phamacology has pointed to a central, rather than to a peripheral, site of action for reserpine, one which many workers consider to be in the hypothalamic area. So far, however, the mode of action of reserpine remains unclear and questions as important as its absorption, its distribution, and its fate within the body—as well as the long latent period before its action—are still unanswered.

The property of reserpine which has aroused the interest of most neuropsychiatrists, and which is chiefly responsible for its reputation in the treatment of mental disorders, consists in a supposedly distinctive sedative action. This differs from the sedative condition associated with barbiturate administration in that while motor activity is subdued, sleep is not induced and the electroencephalographic patterns of sleep are not recorded; further, with human subjects, relief from the distressing emotions associated with states of anxiety, agitation and tension has also been claimed to result from reserpine. It is to such a complex cluster of phenomena that the term *tranquilization* has been applied. According to the Oxford English Dictionary the adjective *tranquil* is defined as "free from agitation or disturbance." Its psychiatric associations, however, are unfortunate, for they hark back to the era of physical restraint and in particular to Benjamin Rush, who in 1835 used the word *tranquilizer* to describe one of his therapeutic instruments. Discussing the "modes of coercion" which might be adopted in the treatment of mania, Rush gave as alternatives:

> confinement by means of a strait waistcoat, or of a chair, which I have called a tranquilizer. He [the patient] submits to them both with less difficulty than to human force, and struggles less to disengage himself from them. The tranquilizer has several advantages over the strait waistcoat or mad shirt. It opposes the impetus of the blood toward the brain, it lessens muscular action everywhere, it reduces the force and frequency of the pulse, it favors the application of cold water and ice to the head, and warm water to the feet . . . it enables the physician to feel the pulse and to bleed without any trouble, or altering the erect position of the patient's body; and lastly, it relieves him, by means of a close stool, half filled with water, over which he constantly sits, from the festor and filth of his alvine evacuations.

Rush's description can claim at least the merit of a clarity missing from the more recent exploitation of this term. In the past three years the epithet *tranquilizing* has been vigorously applied to a number of pharmacologically diverse substances and its metaphorical nature has not always been acknowledged. The word *tranquilizer* is without scientific meaning and should not be employed as a nominal substitute for an understanding of the mode of action of the drug concerned. The need for this knowledge remains unsatisfied, whether the drugs be called "tranquilizers," "ataraxics," "deturmoilizers" or "apatheticatory agents."

It is nonetheless easier to discard the term *tranquilization* than to replace it. Little progress in this direction has been made so far by the many laboratory studies on reserpine. Its actions on the nervous system extend beyond those described to account for its cardiovascular effects and, depending on the investigators' technique, reports have appeared of its action on the limbic system (MacLean et al. 1956), on the midbrain reticular substance (Rinaldi and Himwich 1955), on conditional reflex responses (Gliedmann and Gantt 1956), and on cerebral synaptic transmission (Langfitt et al. 1956). Ingenius biochemical speculations have assigned to reserpine a role as liberator of 5-hydroxytryptramine from binding-sites in the body and brain (Kuntzman et al. 1956). It must be emphasized, however, that even if these physiochemical reactions should be confirmed and elaborated they will remain incomplete without more knowledge of the complementary psychological changes which accompany the response to reserpine.

Interest in psychopharmacology has been reawakened among psychologists in recent years by the carefully controlled operant conditioning techniques associated with the work and views of B. F. Skinner. The chief problem set by these behavioral studies is that of relevance: the effects of reserpine on the pecking responses of pigeons, for example, can be accurately described and repeated but they are difficult to relate to the changes in behavior brought about by reserpine in schizophrenic patients. By contrast, the highly relevant modification of human behavior and experience by pharmacological agents acting on the central nervous system has been systematically studied by very few workers, all of whom agree that the effects produced by these drugs in therapeutic doses depend in part on the personality of the subject and on the circumstances of administration as well as on the physical properties of the drugs (von Felsinger et al. 1955). Very little work of this type has been carried out with reserpine.

In these circumstances reserpine therefore presents a familiar problem to the clinical psychiatrist: namely, that of assessing the efficacy of a therapeutic agent about which too little knowledge has been accumulated in the treatment of conditions whose etiology and natural history are for the most part imperfectly understood. When we began using reserpine at the Maudsley Hospital a few years ago there were very few reliable accounts of its use in the treatment of neuropsychiatric conditions, and almost no controlled clinical studies. Davies and I therefore conducted a clinical trial on a mixed group of outpatients, the majority of whom were suffering from anxiety and depressive reactions. The patients were given either reserpine, prescribed as Serpasil in a dose of 0.5 mg by mouth twice daily, or a seemingly identical placebo, for a period of six weeks. The two substances were allotted by the hospital pharmacist who employed a random method and alone knew the nature of the drug dispensed to each patient; the usual crop of placebo reactions, which was observed during the weekly examinations, quickly demonstrated the importance of such "double-blind" precautions in testing patients of this type.

At the end of the sixth week the response of each patient was estimated by rating scales which were completed by doctors and patients. The results demonstrated a clear-cut difference in favor of those patients treated with reserpine, but it was not possible in a clinical trial of this type to determine which factors would enable the clinician to select or reject individual patients or classes of patients for treatment with the drug (Davies and Shepherd 1955).

An attempt was made to examine the efficacy of reserpine in the treatment of a more homogeneous group: a small number of middle-aged males who presented an indisputable picture of involutional depression and who were reasonably expected to respond to a course of electroconvulsive therapy (ECT). In the treatment of these patients any benefits of drug therapy could be measured against those predicted for a well-tried alternative procedure. The dose of reserpine employed for these patients was much higher than in the prior study, between 10 and 15 mg daily, and was prescribed for three weeks, the period of time during which ECT would otherwise have been administered. No clinical improvement was observed in the patients on reserpine; after a further week without treatment they were started on ECT; all of them recovered after three weeks of this treatment. The value of reserpine in the management of major depressive illness thus appeared dubious; this impression has since been strengthened by the results of Dr. Felix Post's carefully conducted trial of reserpine in the treatment of affective disorders arising in the senium.

The early claims made for reserpine rested on its use in the treatment of chronic mental illness. While the effects of reserpine on a disturbed patient population were being studied at Netherne Hospital, Watt and I studied the response to medication of a group of schizophrenic patients who had resisted all previous treatment and had remained inactive and apathetic for many years (Shepherd and Watt 1956). Twenty-four such patients could be found at St. John's Hospital, Buckinghamshire; all were female, with a mean age of 40.5 years, and a mean hospital stay of 15.8 years. The prognosis was regarded as very poor in every case and a comparison of the effects of reserpine and chlorpromazine on the group was undertaken. The patients were allotted by a random method to three subgroups of eight; a latin square design ensured that each subgroup received reserpine, chlorpromazine, and a placebo over three separate periods of six weeks, originally three times but later twice daily. Regular examinations for side effects and toxicity were made and the patient's clinical state was rated at the end of each six-weekly period. The results indicated that in these conditions chlorpromazine was the drug of choice, not merely because it produced a greater degree of improvement, but principally because the toxic or side effects of reserpine in these doses were much more troublesome. The undesirable effects of the drug included marked restlessness, incontinence of urine and feces, sialorrhea, bulimia, edema of the face, convulsions and, most frequently, a well-marked extrapyramidal syndrome.

The early reports on reserpine emphasized the relatively trivial nature of adverse reactions associated with its use. With the small doses used in the treatment of hypertension, the commonest symptoms—lethargy, nasal obstruction, aching legs, and diarrhea—were not regarded as more than inconvenient. Only when sufficient time had elapsed for therapy to continue for several months was it recognized that a small proportion of hypertensive patients, between 5 percent and 10 percent in most reports, and frequently with a history of previous psychiatric disorder, developed psychiatric symptoms which were usually of a depressive nature and often severe enough to call for ECT (*British Medical Journal* 1955). Larger doses of reserpine have been employed in neuropsychiatric practice, where the wide variation in dose schedule indicates the empirical nature of the treatment. At one extreme 60 mg of reserpine daily have been administered to mental hospital patients (Kinross-Wright 1955), while elsewhere 2–5 mg daily have been considered adequate for comparable populations (Kovitz et al. 1955, Rinaldi et al. 1956). Barsa and Kline (1956) have proposed an initial daily schedule of 5 mg intramuscularly and 3 mg by mouth. The advocates of every reserpine regimen, however, recognize the idiosyncracies and unpredictable responses of individual patients, and modify their doses constantly. During treatment some patients have suffered from an exacerbation of peptic ulcer symptoms and effects, including perforation; the hyperchlorhydria induced by reserpine has been studied experimentally (Schneider and Clark 1956). Convulsions are now also recognized as a complication of treatment, serious enough to contraindicate

ECT during the period of reserpine administration (Foster and Gayle 1955); experimentally, again, reserpine has been shown to lower the seizure threshold in animals (Chen and Ensor 1954).

Other disquieting complications of reserpine treatment which have been reported include cardiac failure, orthostatic collapse, dyspnea, hypothermia and thrombophlebitis, but none of these reactions occurs so frequently during treatment as the group of symptoms which, when fully developed, make up a neurological picture with all the features of postencephalitic Parkinson's disease. While it has been shown that patients who were treated with doses of more than 30 mg of reserpine daily all developed Parkinsonian symptoms (Kinross-Wright 1955), quantity cannot be the sole determining factor in these cases, since some patients react in this way to doses of no more than 5 mg of reserpine daily (Stead and Wing 1955). Whether the neurological symptoms represent inconvenient side effects of reserpine or whether they provide evidence concerning its site of action remains undecided. The recent demonstration that these symptoms can be produced in primates by large doses of reserpine may provide an experimental approach to this question (Windle et al. 1956, Glees and Cole 1956). Since clinical experience meanwhile does not suggest that a favorable response to reserpine is dependent on the appearance of extrapyramidal symptoms, continued administration of the drug beyond the point at which these symptoms develop is inadvisable as long as doubt exists about the possibility of its causing irreversible changes.

Finally, reference should be made to the numerous clinical studies on reserpine which have been reported or are in progress. The drug has been used to treat most of the major psychiatric syndromes as well as conditions as dissimilar as rheumatism, Huntington's chorea and enuresis. The majority of published studies report on the therapeutic results obtained with inpatients. Those which are favorable emphasize that symptomatic improvement, rather than cure, should be expected, but these studies are less precise about the indications for reserpine treatment. Mielke's report from the university clinic at Zurich may be cited as one of the most clinically explicit; on the basis of his experience with nearly four hundred patients he presents the following list of symptoms as provisional indications for reserpine treatment: states of excitement, tension, feelings of unrest, stupor, negativism, mood changes and compulsive drives (Mielke 1956). Other authors have employed nonclinical indices of improvement, such as seclusion rates or the number of ward disturbances. In view of the emphasis on environmental factors that is implicit in the choice of these criteria, little has been done to evaluate the powerful influence of the hospital or ward milieu on the behavior of the patients treated. The interaction between the effects of reserpine and those of a group situation on the organism has been demonstrated experimentally in mice by Christian (1956). At Netherne Hospital, where particular attention has been given to the social aspects of mental hospital life and where reserpine has been administered to socially disturbed patients, the milieu in which treatment was given has proved to be a potent factor in determining the response of patients (*Lancet* 1956, Wing 1956). Observations of this type may help explain the discrepancies in the results obtained with reserpine by workers in different hospitals.

Three questions remain unanswered by the many studies which have been carried out on reserpine. First, whether a particular, self-terminating illness runs a shorter and more satisfactory course than would have been the case if it had been untreated or treated otherwise; second, whether patients with previously intractable mental disease who respond favorably to reserpine do or do not relapse at a later date; and third, whether those patients who are benefited by reserpine treatment differ in an identifiable manner from those who are not. Information of this type is notoriously difficult to obtain about psychiatric outpatients, and an assessment of their response to treatment has been rendered still more difficult by the tendency to combine the administration of reserpine with psychotherapeutic measures. Until these questions can be answered adequately, reserpine will continue to stimulate interest among physiologists, pharmacologists and biochemists working on the central nervous system, but clinicians will suspend judgment about its value as a therapeutic agent.

REFERENCES

Barsa, J. A., and Kline, N. S. (1956). Use of reserpine in disturbed psychotic patients. *American Journal of Psychiatry* 112:684-691.

British Medical Journal (1955). Depression during Rauwolfia therapy. 2:1378.

Chen, G., Ensor, C. R., and Bohner, B. (1954). A facilitation action of reserpine on the central nervous system. *Proceedings of the Society of Experimental Medicine and Biology* 86:507-510.

Christian, J. J. (1956). Reserpine suppression of murine adrenal and reproductive responses to population density. *Federation Proceedings* 15:511.

Cole, J., and Glees, P. (1956). Ritalin as an antagonist to reserpine in monkeys. *Lancet* 1:338.

Davies, D. L., and Shepherd, M. (1955). Reserpine in the treatment of anxious and depressed patients. *Lancet* 2:117-120.

Foster, M. W., and Gayle, R. F. (1955). Dangers in combining reserpine (Serpasil) with electroconvulsive therapy. *Journal of the American Medical Association* 159:1522.

Gliedmann, L. H., and Gantt, W. H. (1956). The effects of reserpine and chlorpromazine on orienting behaviour and retention of conditioned reflexes. *Southern Medical Journal (Birmingham)* 49:880-889.

Kinross-Wright, V. (1955). Chlorpromazine and reserpine in the treatment of psychoses. *Annals of the New York Academy of Sciences* 61:174-182.

Kovitz, B., Carter, J. T., and Addison, W. P. (1955). A comparison of chlorpromazine and reserpine in chronic psychosis. *Archives of Neurology and Psychiatry* 74:467-471.

Kuntzman, R., Udenfriend, E. G., Tomich, E. G., Brodie, B., and Shore, P. A. (1956). Biochemical effect of reserpine on serotomin binding sites. *Federation Proceedings* 15:450.

Lancet (1956). Function of the mental hospital (abstract). 1:485-486.

Langfitt, T. W., Hart, E. R., and Marrazzi, A. S. (1956). Relation between cerebral synaptic actions of mescaline, indoles and tranquilizers. *Federation Proceedings* 15:450-451.

MacLean, P. D., Flanigan, S., Flynn, J. P., Kim, C., and Stevens, J. R. (1956). Hippocampal function: tentative correlations of conditioning, EEG, drug, and radioautographic studies. *Yale Journal of Biology and Medicine* 28:380-395.

Miekle, F. A. (1956). The Rauwolfia alkaloid reserpine (Serpasil) in psychiatry. *Archiv für Psychiatrie und Nervankrankheiten* 194:263.

Rinaldi, F., and Himwich, H. E. (1955). A comparison of effects of reserpine and some barbiturates on the electrical activity of cortical and subcortical structures of the brain of rabbits. *Annals of the New York Academy of Sciences*, pp. 27-35.

Rinaldi, F., Rudy, L. H., and Himwich, H. E. (1956). Clinical evaluation of azacyclonol, chlorpromazine and reserpine on a group of chronic-psychotic patients. *American Journal of Psychiatry* 112:678.

Schneider, E. M., and Clark, M. I. (1956). Hyperchlorhydria induced by intravenous reserpine; response to various therapeutic agents. *American Journal of Digestive Diseases* 1:22-30.

Shepherd, M., and Watt, D. C. (1956). A controlled clinical study of chlorpromazine and reserpine in chronic schizophrenia. *Journal of Neurology, Neurosurgery and Psychiatry* 19:232-235.

Skinner, B. F. (1953). *Science and Human Behavior.* New York: Macmillan.

Stead, J. S., and Wing, J. K. (1955). Parkinsonism during treatment with reserpine. *Lancet* 1:823-824.

von Felsinger, J. M., Lasanga, L., and Beecher, H. K. (1955). Drug induced mood changes in man. 2. Personality and reactions to drugs. *Journal of the American Medical Association* 157:1113-1119.

Windle, W. F., et al. (1956). Akinesia, rigidity, tremor and associated phenomena in reserpinized monkeys and chimpanzees. *Anatomical Record* 124:474.

Wing, L. (1956). The use of reserpine in chronic psychotic patients: a controlled trial. *Journal of Mental Science* 102:530-541.

Chapter 4

The Benzodiazepines as "Anxiolytics"

Despite the accumulation of extensive laboratory data, the precise nature of the pharmacodynamic mode of action of the benzodiazepines remains unclear (Zbinden and Randall 1967). In addition to chlordiazepoxide, diazepam and nitrazepam, two of the other benzodiazepine derivatives in current clinical use also merit mention. Oxazepam ("Seranid-D") is a metabolite of diazepam, with a hydrogen atom replacing the methyl group; medazepam ("Nobrium") resembles diazepam, one of its metabolites, in respect to both chemical structure and pharmacology. Though there is no convincing evidence to suggest that any of these compounds is therapeutically more efficacious than its predecessor, clinical experience shows that individual patients sometimes express a clear preference for one or another of the benzodiazepines.

While the benzodiazepines have been liberally and sometimes indiscriminately used in the treatment of a number of psychiatric and medical conditions, the number of conditions for which their prescription has been specifically established remains relatively small. In the management of epilepsy, diazepam has been widely accepted as a useful anticonvulsant which can be of particular value in the treatment of status epilepticus when administered intravenously. Chlordiazepoxide can be an invaluable drug in treating the alcohol withdrawal syndrome and delirium tremens. Nitrazepam is a relatively safe hypnotic.

It is, however, for their anxiolytic properties that the benzodiazepines have been most widely employed. Their popularity is well attested by prescription figures, especially in general practice. Thus, over the quinquennium 1965-1970 the number of prescriptions for psychotropic drugs in England and Wales increased by 19 percent, much of the rise being attributable to chlordiazepoxide, diazepam and nitrazepam. During this period there was also a clear rise in the consumption of the antidepressant drugs, amitriptyline and imipramine, and a fall in the prescription-rate of barbiturates. In a recent discussion of these trends Parish (1971) concludes: "The increased interest in recognition and treatment of depressive disorders helps to explain the increase in the prescribing of the antidepressant drugs (Tryptizol and Tofranil) but the phenomenal increase in the prescribing of hypnotics (Mandrax and Mogadon) and the minor tranquilizers (Librium and Valium) is difficult to explain."

In view of the importance of psychiatric illness in general practice (Shepherd et al. 1966) there have been surprisingly few attempts to study this prescribing trend in detail, but Parish was able to collect some relevant information from a retrospective analysis of information in the medical records of 48 general practitioners in a single city. In this sample the benzodiazepines proved to be the drugs of choice for "anxiety neurosis," "neurotic depression," and "tension headache," and to figure prominently in the treatment of "affective psychosis," "nervous dyspepsia," and "insomnia." So wide a spectrum of morbidity suggests that the benzodiazepines are being prescribed less for the treatment of specific conditions than as the favored form of medication for what has been called the "alleviation of anxiety in a non-psychotic setting" (*The Medical Letter* 9(2):29, 1969).

The recent history of the rise and fall of meprobamate and its congeners carries clear lessons for overenthusiasm in the use of drugs for the treatment of morbid anxiety. At the present time the evidence from prescription trends indicates that the benzodiazepines are ousting the barbiturates from this role and it would seem to be important to ascertain the relative merits of these two classes of compound before substituting the more recent—and more expensive—alternative for the older drugs, whose advantages and disadvantages are so well known. The two criteria on which such a comparison must be based are efficacy and safety. With regard to the former, the published reports are still inconclusive (Shepherd et al. 1966). Clinical opinion extends from an endorsement of the virtual supersession of the barbiturates by the benzodiazepines to a much more conservative view expressed by some authorities. On the question of safety, however, opinion is much more consistently in favor of the benzodiazepines, chiefly because of the use of barbiturates for suicidal purposes: nitrazepam has, for example, been shown to be a relatively safe hypnotic (Matthew et al. 1969), and very large doses of the benzodiazepines have been ingested without fatality.

But even though they may be relatively safe the benzodiazepines are not free of adverse effects (Shepherd et al. 1972). Tiredness and somnolence are most commonly reported, especially at higher dosage levels. Other well-recognized phenomena are ataxia, headache, vertigo, dizziness, confusion, various autonomic reactions and a paradoxical stimulant effect. Many of these reactions are more pronounced in elderly people. Endocrine disturbances, weight gain and hypersensitivity phenomena are also recorded with use of benzodiazepines, and interference with judgment affecting driving has been observed. The benzodiazepines can potentiate the action of other centrally-acting drugs. It should also be strongly emphasized that they can induce physical dependence, a hazard of potential importance if the drugs are misused (Retterstöl 1971).

In sum, the benzodiazepines may well represent a useful addition to current therapeutics. At present, however, they are probably being overprescribed to an extent which remains to be determined. An adequate explanation of this phenomenon should take account of psychosocial as well as pharmacological factors.

REFERENCES

Matthew, H., Proudfoot, A. T., Aitken, R. C. B., Raeburn, J. A., and Wright, N. (1969). Nitrazepam—a safe hypnotic. *British Medical Journal* 3:23.

Parish, P. A. (1971). The prescribing of psychotropic drugs in general practice. *Journal of the Royal College of General Practitioners* 21 (Supplement 4.) (92):69.

Retterstöl, N. (1971). Birirkninger ar benzodiazepiner. *Nordisk psykiatrisk tidsskrift* 25, 34.

Shepherd, M., Cooper, B., Brown, A. C., and Kalton, G. W. (1966). *Psychiatric Illness in General Practice.* London: Oxford University Press.

Shepherd, M., Lader, M. H., and Lader, S. (1972). Hypnotics and sedatives. In *Side Effects of Drugs,* vol. 7, ed. L. Meyler and

A. Herxheimer, p. 51. Amsterdam: Excerpta Medica Foundation.

The Medical Letter (1969). Librium and Valium. 11 (20).

Zbinden, G., and Randall, L. O. (1967). Pharmacology of benzodiazepines: laboratory and clinical correlations. In *Advances in Pharmacology*, vol. 5, p. 213. New York: Academic Press.

Chapter 5

The Central Action of Psychotropic Drugs

The last ten years have witnessed a growing interest in the place of centrally acting drugs in the treatment of psychiatric illness. The chemist, the pharmacologist and the clinician have been joined by the psychologist in a series of combined operations which have come to be widely known as psychopharmacology. Several large interdisciplinary programs of research into both the action of psychotropic drugs and the responses of the central nervous system to them have been set up with the object of establishing a rational basis for the chemotherapy of mental disorders. If the results so far have been less impressive than those obtained with centrally acting drugs in the therapy of neurological disease, the disparity reflects clinical as well as pharmacological sources of ignorance. It is true that in so well-established a field as that of the treatment of the epilepsies by anticonvulsants Toman (1961) has recently pointed out that "the problems are largely solved by manpower, by empirical methods, by sheer weight of numbers, rather than by theoretical guidelines leading straight to clinical prediction." Even so, the investigator of the better demarcated neurological disorders enjoys two major advantages over his psychiatric colleague: namely a grasp of at least some aspects of pathophysiology and a relatively good correlation between animal and human drug responses.

By contrast, the biological mechanisms of most psychiatric illnesses are still obscure, and clear-cut indices of morbidity against which to measure drug action are often lacking, especially as psychosocial factors must always be included in the assessment of outcome. Furthermore, in the study of the mode of action of psychotropic drugs on higher cerebral functions the extrapolation from animal to man tends to illustrate too often what Roger Russell (1964) refers to as "analogous" rather than "homologous" behavior. In these circumstances it is not surprising that the ingenious maneuvers of the chemist and the behavioral psychologist, allied to a dash of intuitive clinical empiricism, have too often served as substitutes for the experimental investigation of the human pharmacology of these substances. The relatively small number of investigations in this category may be illustrated by three different types of approach.

The first approach exemplifies a traditional method in experimental therapeutics. It depends on the direct transposition to the clinical situation of biological effects ascertained by animal experiment. Perhaps the most cogent application of this approach to psychiatric illness has concerned the action of pharmacological substances employed in the treatment of depressive disorders. The depressive illnesses, it has been claimed, respond to drugs which inhibit the enzyme monoamine oxidase (MAO-inhibitors). Neither the theoretical basis for this claim nor the many clinical trials which have been designed to demonstrate whether or not MAO-inhibitors are effective therapeutic substances are relevant here, however, since most of the clinical experiments with these drugs are indistinguishable from those conducted with empirical remedies. Of greater relevance is the study reported by Pare who, in the context of a double-blind controlled clinical trial, attempted to determine not only whether depressed patients would respond to the drug 1-isonicotinyl-2-isopropylhydrazine (iproniazid), but also: (1) whether those patients who did so respond could be differentiated clinically and biochemically from the nonresponders; and (2) whether the response, when it occurred, could be attributed to change in the brain concentration of 5-HT or the catecholamines (Pare 1959). Biochemical differentiation was undertaken by pretreatment estimates of urinary 5-hydroxyindoleacetic acid in the two patient groups, while attempts to change the concentration of cerebral amines were made by intravenous injections of D,L-5-HTP and DL-DOPA.

Though the results of this experiment were inconclusive they were suggestive enough to encourage another enquiry along similar lines, this time using the MAO-inhibitor N-isonicotinyl (N,N-benzylcarboxamidoethyl) hydrazine, or nialamide, and a more refined biochemical technique: namely, the administration of a loading dose of the enzyme-substrate 5-HT followed by assays of urinary 5-HIAA before and during drug-treatment (Dewhurst and Pare 1961). The purpose of the study was to investigate these biochemical parameters *in vivo* and to correlate them with clinical response. There were wide individual differences in the drop in 5-HIAA excretion following nialamide administration, but an analysis of the individual responses showed no constant relationship between clinical improvement and MAO inhibition. Indeed, in one of the patients whose clinical response to the drug was least equivocal—as confirmed by a relapse on placebo followed by a further response to drug—the change in 5-HT metabolism was least detectable.

A more positive development of this theme has since been reported by Coppen and his coworkers, who have argued that the effects of MAO inhibition on depressed patients should be potentiated by the concurrent administration of tryptophan, the precursor of the two cerebral amines 5-hydroxytryptamine and tryptamine (Coppen et al. 1963). In the course of a four-week double-blind trial with a series of patients receiving the MAO inhibitor tranylcypromine (trans-DL-2-phenylcyclopropylamine), they added tryptophan to the medication during the second week while at the same time a control group received a placebo instead of tryptophan. The bi-weekly ratings of depressive symptoms made during the course of the trial showed that the mean differences from the initial values were significantly higher in the tryptophan-treated group than in their controls (Figure 5-1).

It need hardly be emphasized that any interpretation of the findings in such experiments must still be tentative. For example, since 5-HT does not appear to penetrate the blood-brain barrier, the MAO inhibition observed in the second experiment is presumably peripheral and may or may not correlate with central events. Again, some experimental studies with rats have failed to show a correlation between changes and brain amine levels, so that the theoretical basis of the third experiment remains uncertain (Hess and Doepfuer 1961).

A second approach to confirmatory studies of psychotropic drug effects in man revolves around the application to human behavior of psychological concepts derived from the study of infra-human species. Many of the rather rigid behavioral techniques now so popular as screening-devices fall into this category. Here I would

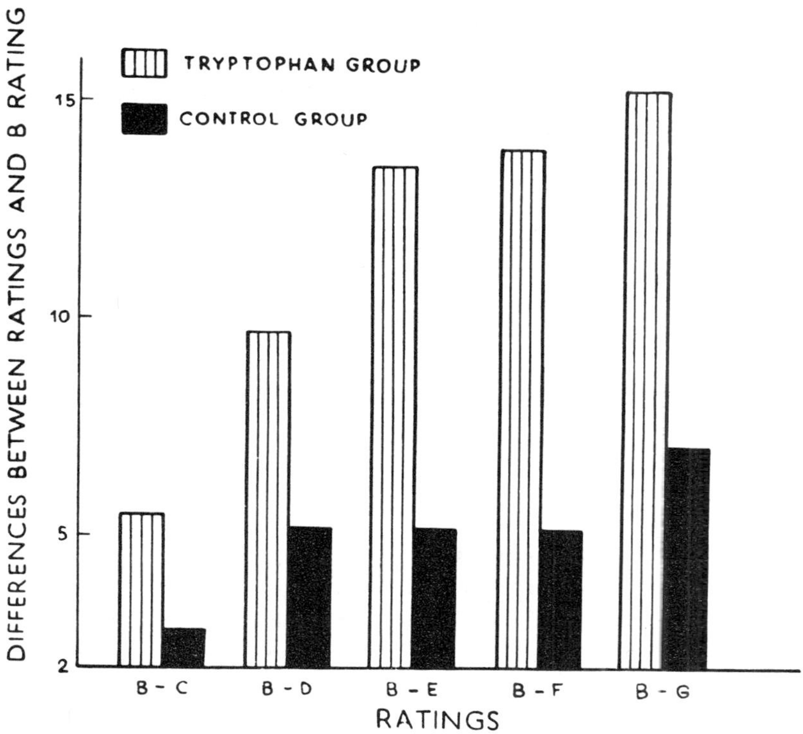

Figure 5-1. Differences between rating B (first week) and successive ratings from the trytophan and control groups. Reprinted with permission from *Lancet* 79 (1963).

refer to the studies of Watt and his co-workers, who have borrowed and developed a suggestion originally advanced by Weiskrantz on the basis of conditioning experiments with monkeys. Weiskrantz suggested that the reserpinized animal's indifference to stimuli in a setting of apparently clear consciousness is dependent on reserpine's property of inducing sensory blockade, leading to what he called "behavioral non-reactivity" (Weiskrantz 1957). This condition would correspond to the crude, nonspecific clinical state of "tranquilization" which, however, could also result from other mechanisms. Watt and Crookes reasoned that if Weiskrantz's hypothesis were correct, the administration of three groups of psychological tests, bearing on the classical triad of sensory, motor, and associational abilities respectively, should lead to evidence of decreased function only in the sensory sphere among human subjects exposed to the action of reserpine (Watt and Crookes 1961). By contrast, another tranquilizer—like chlorpromazine, which possesses quite different neuropharmacological properties—should not exhibit the same psychological correlates. Their original set of experiments indicated: first, that the responses of the reserpinized subjects were in the predicted direction and, second, that they differed radically from those associated with chlorpromazine. Evidence was therefore provided in support of the general hypothesis.

Some of the implications of this concept for abnormal behavior have since been explored by these workers (Allport et al. 1964). They have related the clinical observation that reserpine is often an effective drug in the treatment of mania to their theory of its therapeutic action via the psychological phenomenon of distractability. This symptom arises in part from the disturbance of the manic patient's capacity to discriminate relevant from irrelevant aspects of the total sensory input. Prominent among selective sensory mechanisms of the normal brain is sensory adaptation or *satiation*. A process closely related to Hull's reactive inhibition, its function is to filter out information of low uncertainty from the healthy central nervous system so that a smooth inflow of sensory stimuli can be regulated. In mania, satiation is excessive; consequently, the patient suffers from an oversuppression of sensory input—a process which, according to theory, leads to distractability as a form of compensatory behavior. If, therefore, reserpine reduced sensory input, its therapeutic action in mania should be linked to its ability to reduce satiation. Accordingly, three tests of satiation were administered to sixteen subjects, all of whom had received reserpine during the previous four weeks. Over the ensuing two weeks half the group continued to receive the drug, the other half received a placebo. The results are depicted in Figure 5-2.

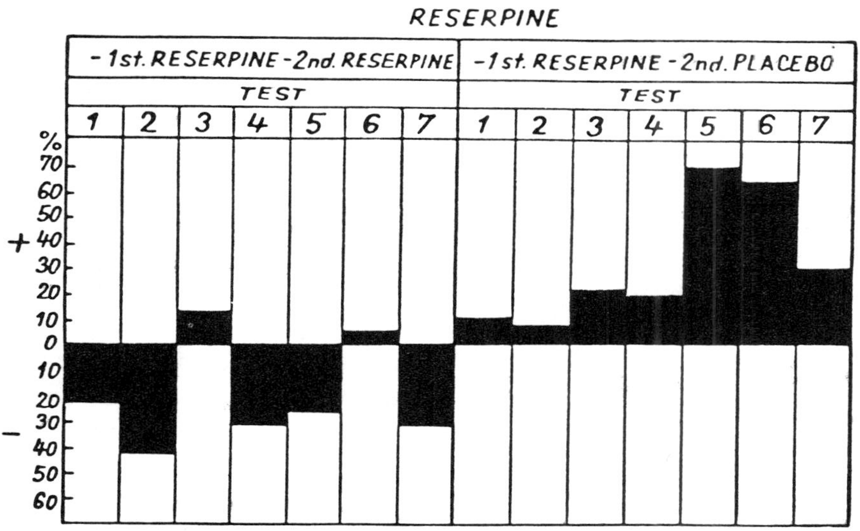

Figure 5-2. Satiation tests. Key: + = Increased satiation on second test. Tests: 1, Spiral after-effect; 2, Figure-ground reversals, spontaneous rate; 3, Figure-ground reversals, minimum rate; 4, Figure-ground reversals, maximum rate; 5, Binocular rivalry, spontaneous rate; 7, Binocular rivalry, maximum rate. Reprinted with permission from Bradley, Flugel, and Hoch (1964).

From these results it is apparent that, in accordance with prediction, the seven measures derived from the three tests indicate a decrease in satiation among those subjects who continued to receive reserpine; the indices of satiation, on the contrary, were significantly raised when placebo was administered. To this extent, therefore, the hypothesis was confirmed.

The third approach takes its starting point from the differences between the drug-responses of normal human subjects and those of psychiatric patients. Investigations of this type depend on the prior establishment of clear-cut parameters distinguishing the two groups, a difficult objective to attain with many mental illnesses. At the Institute of Psychiatry and University College, London, a small team of workers has been tackling the problem of morbid anxiety and autonomic dysfunction from this standpoint. From this work I have selected one set of experiments conducted by Dr. Malcolm Lader.

The patients were all suffering from affective reactions with morbid anxiety as the dominant symptom. Normal subjects matched for sex and age were used as controls. Both patients and controls were examined under identical, standardized laboratory conditions. Both were left undisturbed for 10 minutes before 20 auditory stimuli—standardized at 100 decibels in volume, 100 cycles-per-second in frequency, and 1 second in duration—were applied automatically and in random sequence at intervals ranging from 45 to 85 seconds.

The electrical resistance of the skin has been shown by Lader and Montagu (1962) to be dependent on a cholinergic mechanism and hence to reflect sweat gland activity. Three aspects of sweat gland activity, as measured by the skin resistance method, were studied: they were the level of activity, the rate of habituation, and spontaneous fluctuations in the level of activity. After the initial testing, the patients were placed on either placebo or sodium amytal for one week; in the subsequent week, in a balanced crossover design, they received the alternative treatment. At the end of each week, the physiological tests were repeated. Clinical assessments were also undertaken and a self-rating scale, based on symptoms, was administered to all subjects.

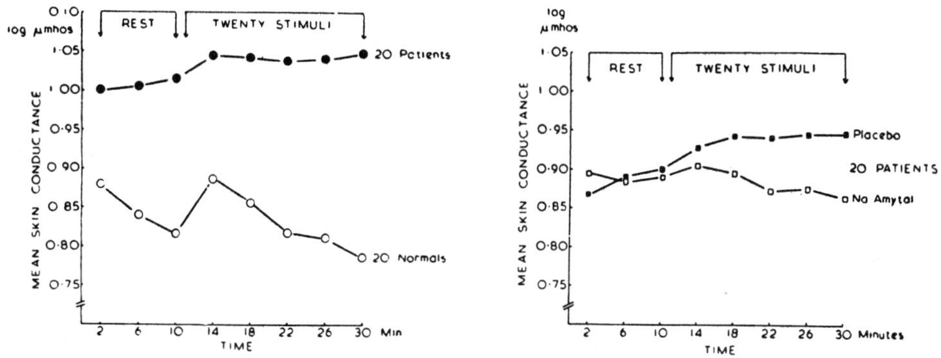

Figure 5-3. Skin conductance.

First, it is clear from Figure 5-3 that the level of sweat gland activity throughout the experimental situation tended to rise in the patient group and to drop in the normal group. The administration of 1 grain of sodium amytal three times daily to the patients, however, changed their sweat gland activity in the direction of the normal pattern. Second, the responses are seen in Figure 5-4 to have diminished more rapidly (i.e., the rate of habituation was greater) in the normals than in the patients, while the barbiturate accelerated habituation in the anxious subjects (the responses are plotted against a logarithmic time scale in order to give a rectilinear decay). Third, although spontaneous fluctuations in the sweat gland activity of the patients are seen in Figure 5-5 to have been more frequent than those of the normal subjects, the number of fluctuations was lowered by the drug. Since all of the differences depicted are significant beyond the 1 percent level of probability, the general effect of barbiturate on each measure was, therefore, to "normalize" the pattern of response in accordance with clinical observations.

Following-up these results, Lader has proceeded to take one variable from each of the three measures and has combined these statistically to yield that function which discriminated best between the normal subjects and the anxious patients. The discriminant function scores are shown in Figure 5-6. A fair discrimination was attained (only three subjects were misclassified), and when the physiological scores for the fifteen patients with morbid anxiety as a largely isolated symptom were plotted against the clinical observers' independent rating of "free-floating anxiety" immediately before the physiological recording, a significant rank-order correlation of 0.93 was obtained. This finding suggests that a physiological index of this type, related as it is to sudomotor sympathetic discharge, may prove to be a useful predic-

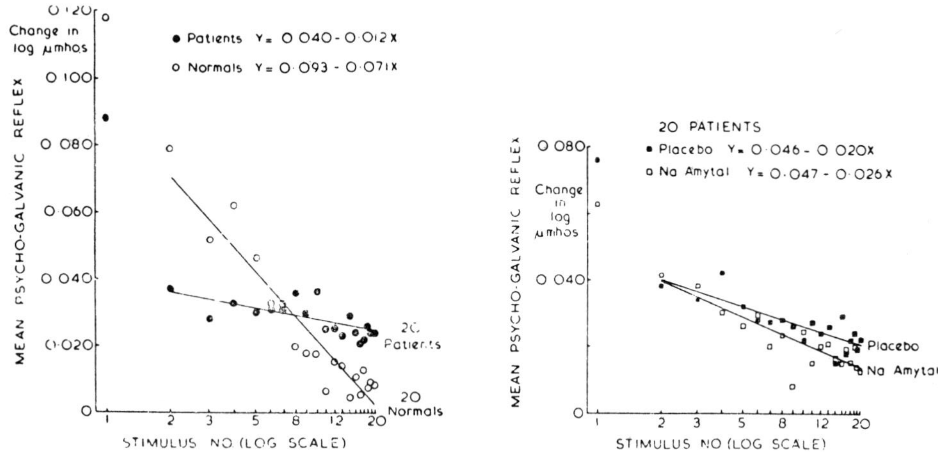

Figure 5-4. The habituation of the psycho-galvanic reflex.

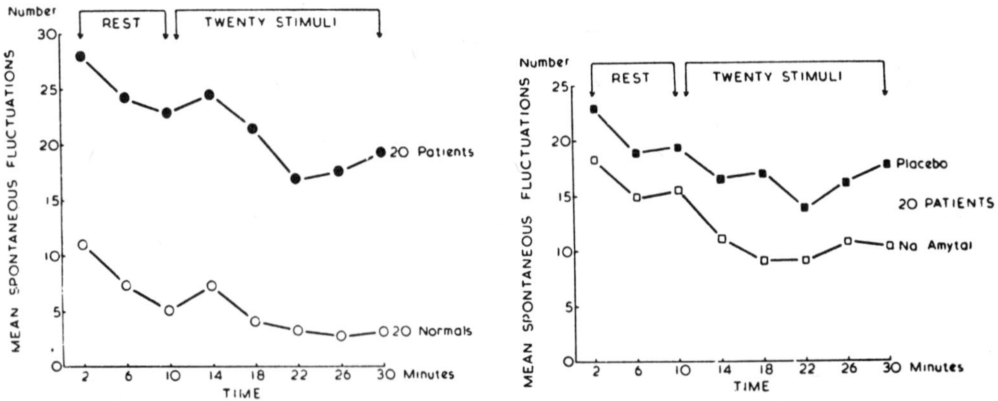

Figure 5-5. Skin conductance fluctuations.

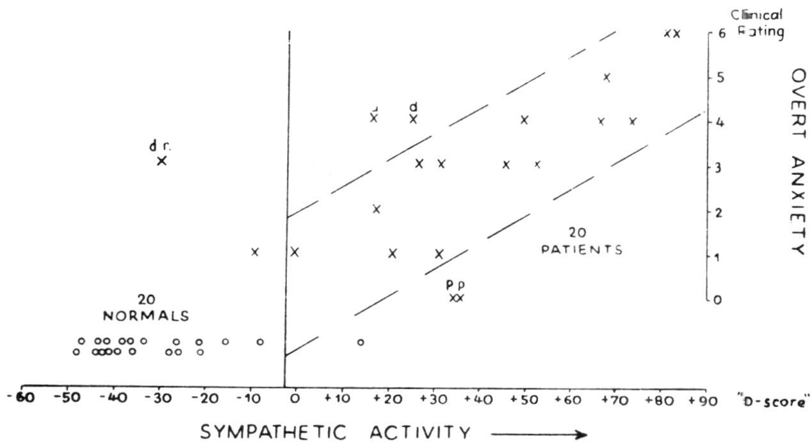

Figure 5-6. A physiological index, related to sudomotor sympathetic discharge.

tor of the degree of clinically-defined anxiety as displayed by the patient under experimental conditions. If this is confirmed, Lader's technique makes it possible to obtain quantitative measures of sedative-drug action, so that formal pharmacological procedures—such as bioassay—can be attempted. A bioassay of Librium against sodium amytal, using two doses of each drug, was then carried out.

All three sets of experiments exemplify the use of human pharmacology in the investigation of centrally acting substances. They share the merit of a rational approach to an understanding of the action of psychotropic drugs in man and, eventually, to the chemotherapy of psychiatric illness.

REFERENCES

Allport, D. A., Crookes, T. G., and Watt, D. C. (1964). The effects of reserpine and chlorpromazine on stimulus-satiation and distractability in human subjects. In *Neuropsychopharmacology,* vol. 3, eds. P. Bradley, F. Flugel, and P. Hoch,p. 42. Amsterdam: Elsevier.

Coppen, A., Shaw, D. M., and Farrell, J. P. (1963). Potentiation of the antidepressive effect of a monoamine-oxidase inhibitor by tryptophan. *Lancet* 1:79.

Dewhurst, W. G., and Pare, C. M. B. (1961). A clinical and biochemical study of monoamine oxidase inhibition in depressed patients. *Journal of Mental Sciences* 107:244.

Hess, S. M., and Doepfuer, W. (1961). Behavioural effects and brain amine content in rats. *Archives Internationales de Pharmacodynamie et Therapie* 134:89.

Lader, M. H., and Montagu, J. D. (1962). The psycho-galvanic reflex: a pharmacological study of the peripheral mechanism. *Journal of Neurology, Neurosurgery, and Psychiatry* 25:126.

Pare, C. M. B. (1959). Iproniazid in the treatment of depression. *Proceedings of the Royal Society of Medicine* 52:585.

Russell, R. W. (1964). Extrapolation from animals to man. In *Animal Behaviour and Drug Action*, eds. H. Steinberg, A. de Rueck, and J. Knight, p. 40. London: J.A. Churchill, Ltd.

Toman, J. E. P. (1961). Pharmacologic problems in evolving new drugs in the field of neurologic and sensory diseases. In *Evaluation of Drug Therapy*, ed. F. M. Forster, p. 17. Madison: University of Wisconsin Press.

Watt, D. C., and Crookes, T. G. (1961). The effect of reserpine on perceptual performance in human subjects. In *Neuropsychopharmacology*, vol. 2, ed. E. Rothlin. Amsterdam: Elsevier.

Weiskrantz, L. (1957). Reserpine and behavioural non-reactivity. In *Psychotropic Drugs*, ed. S. Garattini and V. Ghetti, p. 67. Amsterdam: Elsevier.

Chapter 6

Psychotropic Drug Interactions

The problems of drug interaction interest—or should interest—clinical psychiatrists for three principal reasons. In the first place, they are perhaps more familiar than most clinicians with the issues posed by the general notion of interaction, partly as a statistical concept and partly as a key variable in therapeutics. Furthermore, since biological, psychological and social factors all play some part in the causation and outcome of most mental illness, clinical psychiatrists have, or should have, learned to appreciate that it is unwise to view any one therapeutic measure in isolation. And having grasped the importance of interaction between drug therapy and the milieu in which it is administered (Shepherd 1964) they are unlikely to disregard interaction within its narrower, biological field. Second, since polypharmacy, and its attendant dangers, accompany clinical ignorance, they can be expected to be rife in a branch of medicine where so much remains to be learned. Third, psychiatric patients include addicts whose large appetites for drugs afford opportunity for the observation of toxic and other adverse drug reactions.

In themselves, however, these factors lead principally to a concern with what Schwartz and Lazar (1964) refer to as *empirical*, as distinct from *explanatory*, drug interaction. Empirical interaction, as they point out, can do no more than compare the results obtained by each investigator separately. The problems here are practical: the raw data are observational and may be difficult to interpret. With explanatory interaction, on the other hand, the clinician can hope to make predictions and employ generalizations drawn from biological mechanisms. In this sphere, and at the present time, the direct contribution of the pharmacologist to our knowledge of centrally-acting substances appears to be limited.

Sir John Gaddum (1961), for example, arguing that the most profitable approach to antagonism between centrally-acting drugs will depend on experiments in which indirect effects are excluded, has advocated the study of impulse transmission through one particular synapse to which drugs might be applied by ionophoresis. Perhaps he is right but we are unlikely to see clinical results from this in the near future. Meanwhile, we do know something about the complexity of the empirical laws governing drug interaction from the elegant demonstrations of the late Walter Loewe, whose isobolograms are best visualized in three dimensions. Loewe's work pays due regard to the multiple effects of single drugs in animals but it has been applied very little to human subjects and hardly at all to the human central nervous system (Goodman 1964).

Clearly, the scientific map of psychotropic drug interactions is still largely uncharted. I propose, therefore, to refer to a few expeditions in human and clinical pharmacology, chosen as much to underline method as to illustrate achievement.

First, there are two experiments which employ orthodox pharmacological reasoning to study explanatory interactions, a procedure rare enough in psychopharmacology. The first was centered on amphetamine, a sympathomimetic amine which has been used extensively in psychiatric practice with very little understanding of its central actions in man. In view of the evidence suggesting that the peripheral actions of amphetamine might be related to noradrenaline release, this drug was administered intravenously to normal human subjects who had previously ingested large doses of reserpine in order to deplete their stores of catecholamines (Gelder and Vane 1962). The subjects' blood pressure was taken as the principal index of peripheral responses in a preliminary control period, and psychological reactions, rated by subject and observer, constituted a guide to the central action of the drug. The reserpinized subjects who had failed to demonstrate the normal, short-lived hypersensitive response to an intravenous injection of 10 mg of tyramine—presumably as a result of the depletion of noradrenaline stores by reserpine—nonetheless responded to amphetamine in the usual way. Furthermore, following the administration of amphetamine the characteristic malaise exhibited by all the reserpinized subjects was abruptly terminated and replaced by the mildly euphoric reaction that had been reported in the control period. Seemingly, therefore, neither the peripheral nor the central actions of amphetamine was impaired, and it seems unlikely that either could depend on an intermediary release of noradrenaline as the mode of action for this drug.

The second experiment has to do with imipramine. It depends on the observation that in rats and mice the reserpine-syndrome—consisting of hypothermia, profound sedation, muscular rigidity and miosis—can be inhibited and even reversed by the administration of imipramine. This same action is also exhibited by antidepressant drugs related chemically to imipramine, which interact in a similar way with benzoquinolizine derivatives, whose effects are similar to those of reserpine. Since the therapeutic action of the tricyclic antidepressants has not yet been clearly associated with any one of their pharmacological properties, and since these drugs appear to exercise relatively trivial effects on normal humans, it seemed reasonable to enquire whether their anti-reserpine and anti-benzoquinolizine actions might not be taken to reflect their antidepressant action, especially as reserpine is known to induce morbid depression in clinical practice.

For this purpose a group of normal volunteer subjects received intramuscular injections of tetrabenazine followed by an injection of desmethylimipramine (DMI) or placebo (Dick and Shepherd 1965). The effects of tetrabenazine were determined by a series of psychophysiological measurements and a specially constructed questionnaire. The results analyzed so far suggest that on some of these indices desmethylimipramine counteracted the initial effect of tetrabenazine. If these results are confirmed, a pharmacological interaction of this type might constitute a useful model both for testing certain new drugs on normal subjects and for studying the physiopathological mechanisms of depressive states.

Here, then, are two attempts to explore explanatory interactions which are of obvious clinical relevance. At the same time it should be emphasized that in the clinic, where he is as much concerned with behavioral phenomena as with physiochemical mechanisms, the psychiatrist *qua* clinician encounters chiefly empirical interactions. Clinical drug effects are assessed, initially at least and often crudely enough, in behavioral terms.

The scientific evaluation of behavior in the field of psychotropic drug interaction, however, has proved a difficult exercise even in the case of what has probably been the most intensively studied example, namely the interaction between alcohol and the barbiturates. Animal studies have yielded conflicting reports on the question of whether these substances produce additive or synergistic effects (Gruber 1955). There have been individual case reports suggesting fatalities due to their mutual potentiation (Jetter and McLean 1943), but in view of the huge annual consumption of both alcohol and barbiturates it is evident that a high mortality rate is unlikely to be a significant consequence of their interaction. When death occurs in humans it is more likely to be a secondary phenomenon resulting from impairment of the psychomotor coordination necessary for driving a vehicle. It has been maintained that a number of drugs, including isoniazid, azidepyrine, the antihistamines, the opiates, the urea derivatives and the sulfonamides can intensify the noxious effects of alcohol and so affect driving abilities adversely (Lickint 1956). A rigorous demonstration of these interaction effects on human behavior, however, depends on studies like those of Joyce and his colleagues, who have investigated the potentiation of ethyl alcohol by phenobarbital on standardized tasks under laboratory conditions (Joyce et al. 1959). Such studies are unfortunately still uncommon, depending as they do on the active collaboration of psychologists prepared to work both experimentally with human subjects and to pay due regard to pharmacological principles.

Another approach to the problem of drug-alcohol interactions has come from Goldberg, who has shown with electro-onlographic techniques that horizontal positional nystagmus and horizontal roving ocular movements both occur as aftereffects of drinking, and continue after alcohol has been eliminated from the bloodstream (Goldberg 1961). These responses and their distressing subjective correlates—which include the "hangover"—are demonstrably modified by centrally-acting drugs administered with the original dose of alcohol.

The most direct and dramatic clinical studies of alcohol-barbiturate interactions, however, have been those carried out on volunteer addicts at the United States Public Health Service Addiction Center at Lexington, Kentucky. In these, the essential similarity of the clinical picture following sudden withdrawal of large doses of either alcohol or barbiturates was first established (Wikler 1964). This so-called abstinence syndrome consists of weakness, tremulousness, anorexia, insomnia, convulsions and delirium. In the Lexington study, an attempt was made to induce it by first withdrawing one drug and then to control it by administering the other. In this way it was possible to demonstrate a partial equivalence between the alcohol and the barbiturate, which in turn has suggested that the well-tried clinical practice of treating the alcoholic abstinence syndrome with cerebral depressants might be regarded as a form of substitution therapy.

The principles of the above, relatively crude clinical experiment have been refined quantitatively by Isbell and his colleagues (1959). Their starting point has been the similar physical effects and subjective responses obtained with the two psychotomimetic drugs, LSD–25 and psilocybin. Using a crossover design with subjects acting as their own controls, these workers have shown that direct tolerance to both LSD and psilocybin can be developed, and also that subjects rendered tolerant to one drug are cross-tolerant of the other (Isbell et al. 1961). Other experiments have demonstrated a similar relationship between LSD–25 and mescaline, so that evidence exists for cross-tolerance between drugs of similar action but different chemical structure. This indicates that such drugs either share a common biological mechanism or a common final pathway (Wolbach et al. 1962).

The preceding notion opens up so many possibilities of interaction between centrally acting drugs that caution might be expected to be the rule in the manufacture and prescription of drug-combinations. Unfortunately, this is not the case. Among such combinations those containing amphetamines and barbiturates are probably the most popular. There are now several such preparations available, enough to render the so-called "purple heart" problem a matter of pharmacological interest as well as of public health concern. Yet only recently, long after we have known that they are associated with addictive, toxic, psychotic and antisocial phenomena, are we beginning to learn a little about the action of amphetamine-barbiturate combinations. It has been left to Steinberg and her colleagues (Rushton and Steinberg 1964) to show not only that the effects of mixtures of amobarbital and amphetamine on rats' exploratory behavior in a Y-maze are in excess of those produced by individual or additive doses of either drug, but that similar differences can be demonstrated with normal human subjects as well. Using amphetamine sulfate and cyclobarbital in two different ratios, one approximating that employed in the commercial preparation "Drinamyl," the other with a much higher proportion of the barbiturate, these workers have suggested that the effects of the mixtures on pulse-rate, simple tasks and subjective responses differ from those of their individual constituents, and that of the two combinations the one containing the lower dosage of barbiturate was preferable (Dickens et al. 1965).

Insofar as empirical studies of this type lend experimental support to clinical practice, they are valuable in their own right. Thus it is much to be regretted that so few comparable studies have been conducted on proprietary mixtures of amphetamine with other substances, or on combinations of the newer psychotropic drugs. It may be that a carefully adjusted combination of a "rapid-acting antidepressant" and a "versatile tranquilizer" together "restore the normal resiliency of mood"; or that it is possible to both lift depression and calm anxiety by the joint action of two drugs of which neither alone is of proven value in the treatment of morbid anxiety or depression. The evidence remains to be produced. Similarly, the claim that two phenothiazines are better than one for the control of major psychoses appears to be based largely on asseveration: I know of only one clinical experiment which purports to test this hypothesis (Talbot 1964).

Finally, no survey of this subject can nowadays be complete without a word about the adverse effects of drug interaction, which can constitute significant starting points of scientific enquiry. The monoamine oxidase inhibitors are known to interact adversely with several compounds and the Committee on Safety of Drugs already has a list of adverse reactions reported in association with the combined use of other antidepressants with phenothiazines during the first few months of reporting. It is not yet possible to assess the significance of these associations at this early stage, but the system potentially opens up important prospects for the future. It is evident that clinical observation has much to offer provided that the observation is systematic and that the frequency as well as the quality of responses can be estimated. For example, anesthetists, who premedicate their patients with psychotropic drugs (McNaught et al. 1965), have reported that after the administration of phenothiazines there was during anesthesia a potentiation of pethidine, a liability to hypotension and a marked pallor; postoperatively they mention prolonged unconsciousness, hypotension and pallor. Since drug consumption has come to constitute one of the distinguishing characteristics of the modern psychiatric patient the possibilities of a drug-monitoring program in defined populations (Finney 1965) could be profitably explored in this field. It is potentially a rewarding as well as an onerous task for the future.

REFERENCES

Dick, P., and Shepherd, M. (1965). A study of the interaction between desmethylimipramine and tetrabenazine in normal man. *Psychopharmacologia* 8:32-40.

Dickins, D. W., Lader, M. H., and Steinberg, H. (1965). Differential effects of 2 amphetamine-barbiturate mixtures in man. *British Journal of Pharmacology* 24:14-23.

Finney, D. J. (1965). The design and logic of a monitor of drug use. *Journal of Chronic Diseases* 18:77-98.

Gaddum, J. H. (1961). Antagonisms between drugs. In *Neuropsychopharmacology*, vol. 2, ed. E. Rothlin, pp. 19-24. Amsterdam: Elsevier.

Gelder, M. G., and Vane, J. R. (1962). Interaction of the effects of tyramine, amphetamine and reserpine in man. *Psychopharmacologia* 3:231-241.

Goldberg, L. (1961). Alcohol, tranquilizers and hangover. *Quarterly Journal of Studies on Alcohol*. Supplement No. 1:37-56.

Goodman, L. (1964). In *Drugs in Our Society*, ed. P. Talslay, p. 49. Baltimore: Johns Hopkins Press.

Gruber, C. M., Jr. (1955). A theoretical consideration of additive and potentiated effects between drugs with a practical example using alcohol and barbiturates. *Archives Internationales de Pharmacodynamie et de Therapie* 102:17-32.

Isbell, H. (1959). Comparison of the reactions induced by psilocybin and LSD-25 in man. *Psychopharmacologia* 1:29-38.

Isbell, H., Wolbach, A. B., Wikler, A., and Milner, E. J. (1961). Cross tolerance between LSD and psilocybin. *Psychopharmacologia* 2:147-159.

Jetter, W., and McLean, R. (1943). Poisoning by synergistic effect of phenobarbital and ethyl alcohol: experimental study. *Archives of Pathology* 36:112-122.

Joyce, C. R. B., Edgecombe, P. C. E., Kennard, D. A., Weatherall, M., and Woods, D. P. (1959). Potentiation by phenobarbitone of effects of ethyl alcohol on human behaviour. *Journal of Mental Science* 105:51-60.

Lickint, F. (1956). *Suchtgefahren* (Hamburg), 1, 1.

McNaught, Inglis J., and Barrow, M. E. H. (1965). Premedication—a reassessment. *Proceedings of the Royal Society of Medicine* 58:29-32.

Rushton, R., and Steinberg, H. (1964). Modification of behavioural effects of drugs by past experience. In *Animal Behavior and Drugs*, ed. H. Steinberg, A. V. S. de Reuck, and J. Knight, pp. 207-223. London: Churchill.

Schwartz, D., and Lazar, P. (1964). Interactions biologiques. *Revue Francaise des Etudes Cliniques et Biologiques* 9:592.

Shepherd, M. (1964). Effectiveness of drugs in relationship to psychological and social forms of treatment. In *Neuropsychopharmacology*, vol. 3, ed. P. B. Bradley, F. Flugel, and P. Hoch, pp. 139-142. Amsterdam, Elsevier.

Talbot, D. R. (1964). Are tranquilizer combinations more effective than a single tranquilizer? *American Journal of Psychiatry* 121:597-600.

Wikler, A. (1964). Introduction. In *Proceedings of the Twenty-Sixth International Congress of Alcoholism*, Stockholm, p. 3.

Wolbach, A. B., Isbell, H., and Miner, E. J. (1962). Cross tolerance between mescaline and LSD reactions. *Psychopharmacologia* 3:1-14.

Part II

Therapeutic Evaluation

Chapter 7

The Evaluation of Psychiatric Remedies

The relatively short history of modern psychiatry has witnessed the rise and fall of many different forms of treatment. At the present time few branches of medicine stand more in need of reliable methods for the assessment of their therapeutic claims. If this unsatisfactory state of affairs springs in some measure from an uncertainty about the causes and nature of most psychiatric illness it also reflects a failure on the part of many workers to have applied to psychiatry well-recognized principles of clinical investigation. Since the establishment of the Therapeutic Trials Committee of the British Medical Research Council in 1931, a number of studies in other medical fields have demonstrated the value of collaboration between the clinician, the statistician, the laboratory scientist and, more recently, the clinical pharmacologist. The combined skills of these specialists have shaped and developed the modern controlled clinical trial, a procedure which has been defined as "an experiment carried out with the object of seeing whether a treatment has any effect on the course of a disease" (Doll 1965).

It should be emphasized at the outset that in its fully developed form the clinical trial takes its place as the cornerstone of the late confirmatory stage of therapeutic evaluation. The stage of early evaluation calls for more empirical procedures which may have to be uncontrolled and in some measure intuitive. In the case of the drug treatment of mental illness, for example, a report from the World Health Organization suggests that the early evaluation stage be subdivided into two phases, the first concerned with dose-range, side effects and toxic reactions, and the second with therapeutic range and effectiveness (World Health Organization 1967). Only in the third phase of therapeutic evaluation are strictly controlled techniques employed, ideally in an attempt to validate the observations already made in the two earlier stages. In the field of psychiatry, there have been very few attempts to explore the early stages of evaluation, and formal clinical trials have suffered in consequence (Blackwell and Shepherd 1967).

In principle, the clinical trial consists in comparing the outcome of two identical groups differing only by virtue of the remedy which one of them receives (see Figure 7-1). The logic of the controlled, or comparative, clinical trial is therefore clearest when its aim is prophylactic; as for example, when attack rates are estimated after the vaccination of populations which are initially free of disease and, therefore, theoretically homogenous. When the population is already diseased the comparative trial may not always be necessary: for example, an untreated illness may carry a one hundred percent mortality rate, or the effectiveness of a new treatment may be so dramatic as to be self-evident. In general, the controlled trial is likely to be most valuable when rational treatment is administered to a clearly defined disorder of known etiology whose outcome can be established by unequivocal criteria. Excellent models have been provided by the treatment of several acute bacterial infections and of some chronic physical illnesses (e.g. pulmonary tuberculosis), whose nature and course are well understood. Such conditions, however, do not apply to most instances of physical disease, nor to virtually any psychiatric disorders. Here, the primary question is not so much whether a particular treatment is effective, but rather how it compares in efficacy with some alternative. With chronic physical disease of obscure etiology and uncertain outcome, for instance, the comparative trial encounters difficulties that are essentially similar to those arising in the treatment of most psychiatric disorders. These issues may be considered conveniently by a brief discussion of some of the principal problems posed by the investigation.

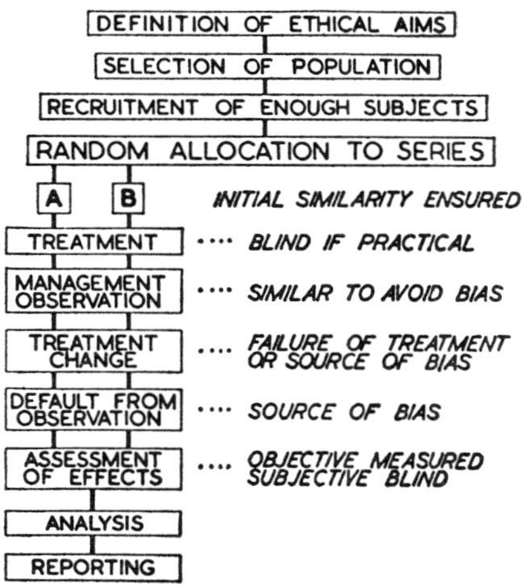

Figure 7-1. Essentials of a comparative trial. Reprinted with permission from Sainsbury and Kreitman (1975).

ETHICS

Although the ethical aspects of the clinical trial in psychiatry in no way differ from those that apply to other forms of illness, the burden is lightened to some extent by the small number of established remedies. Thus, while the psychiatric patient should not suffer by having effective treatment withheld for more than a limited period of time, experience in this branch of medicine suggests that the moral imperative should as likely be exercised against the over-treatment of mental disease, especially when the patient's symptoms impair his capacity for rational communication or affect his ability to participate freely in the therapeutic procedure. The physical treatment of psychiatric illness has provided some unfortunate examples of therapeutic zeal in the past, and newer fashions in pharmacotherapy have already illustrated the dangers of administering compounds with uncertain properties in large quantities over long periods of time.

Some clinicians have adduced ethical arguments for trying to avoid the use of controlled therapeutic experiments. A characteristic example may be taken from the current vogue for the supposedly prophylactic use of lithium carbonate in the management of depressive illnesses. Two of the advocates of this practice write as follows: "Since a striking prophylactic action of lithium became apparent with the first patient studied, it would have been difficult as well as painful to distribute the patients into two groups, one to receive lithium and one to be given placebo or the traditional, and in most cases rather ineffective, therapy. Since prophylactic rather than therapeutic effects were studied, the patients—many of them severely handicapped by frequent relapses—would have had to remain in their group for a number of years" (Baastrup and Schou 1967).

The response to this mode of reasoning has been clearly stated by Pickering (1960): "All therapy is experimentation. Because what in fact we are doing is to alter one of the conditions, or perhaps more than one, under which our patient lives. This is the very nature of an experiment, because an experiment is a controlled observation in which one alters one or more variables at a time to try and see what happens. The difference between haphazard therapy and a controlled clinical trial is that in haphazard therapy we carry out experiments without design on our patients, and therefore our experiments are bad experiments from which it is impossible to learn. The controlled clinical trial means merely introducing the ordinary accepted criteria of a good scientific experiment."

In practice, while each case must be treated on its merits, every investigator concerned with the problems of therapeutic evaluation can profitably address himself to the six questions posed by Bradford Hill (1963), who has played a major role in the development of the modern clinical trial.

1. Is the proposed treatment safe or, in other words, is it likely to do harm to the patient?
2. Can a new treatment be ethically withheld from a new patient in the doctor's care?
3. What patients may be brought into a controlled trial and allocated randomly to different treatments?
4. Is it necessary to obtain the patient's consent to his inclusion in a controlled trial?
5. Is it ethical to use a placebo or dummy treatment?
6. Is it proper for the doctor not to know the treatment being administered to his patient?

CONSTRUCTION OF PATIENT POPULATION

The guiding principles of this phase of the investigation have been expounded clearly by Hill (1960): "In a simple experiment in the laboratory the scientific worker wishes to see what happens to A if he manipulates B. He tries to keep constant all other factors that may upset or influence the relationship. Similarly in the controlled trial we endeavor to keep constant the characteristics of those on treatment A and those on treatment B. Some of those characteristics we can keep constant by stratification—by keeping equal in the two groups such obvious features as age and sex. Other characteristics we cannot deliberately equalize and our aim is to achieve it by the random allocation which, in the long run, offers no favor to one or other group."

The securing of homogeneity in groups of diseased subjects is greatly facilitated by knowledge of the etiology and course of the illness concerned. In a Medical Research Council trial of the treatment of tuberculosis by streptomycin, for example, it was possible to define succinctly the patients entering the trial as suffering from "acute progressive bilateral pulmonary tuberculosis, believed to be of recent origin, bacteriologically proved, unsuitable for collapse therapy, age group 15-30." By contrast, the clinical criteria for inclusion in the first Medical Research Council trial of therapy in depressive illness could not be defined more objectively than in the following terms: "The clinical features of the illness must reveal as its primary manifestations a persistent alteration of mood exceeding customary sadness and constituting a major symptom of the illness. This should be supported by one or more of the following symptoms: self-depreciation with a morbid sense (or delusional ideas) of guilt; sleep disturbance; hypochondriasis; retardation of thought and action; agitated behavior" (Medical Research Council 1965).

Diagnostic categories that depend on such uncertain criteria are open to large observer variation. Furthermore, psychiatric populations defined in these terms are inevitably heterogeneous: in consequence, it is imperative to recruit sufficient numbers of subjects in each group for random allocation, in order to equalize bias. For this reason it may prove necessary to organize a multi-center trial, a complex undertaking which demands considerable time and resources.

BIAS

When treatment has been instituted bias may arise from several sources. After the random allocation of patients there may be changes of treatment or dropouts in the course of therapy, both of which may distort the composition of the patient groups significantly. Such factors can be minimized by careful attention to practical management. Another major bias, however, may be introduced by the expectations of the medical attendant and the patient. This is a matter of particular importance in the management of many psychiatric conditions, where subjective factors enter so intimately into the nature of the illnesses and their outcomes. In these circumstances the double-blind technique, designed to keep the observer and the patient in ignorance of the treatment prescribed, can be valuable. It is important to stress, however, that this technique may be inapplicable when:(1) a drug has detectable side effects, (2) when a placebo must not be administered for ethical reasons, or (3) when the nature of the therapeutic procedure cannot be disguised (Rickels et al. 1970).

THE CRITERIA OF RESPONSE

Inasmuch as the objectives of any treatment must be defined before its success can be estimated, psychiatric illnesses have in the past suffered by comparison with physical illnesses. Zubin (1953) has underlined the reason for this as follows:

In the case of physical disorders the goal of therapy is usually self-evident. The corresponding goal in mental disorder is more difficult to define since we do not know the level to which the patient is to be returned. Should it be to his premorbid level; should it be to the level which he is capable of attaining when one takes into consideration the disease process and its after effects; or should it be to the average level of the general population who never had the illness? The following criteria have been proposed by various workers for gauging the goals of therapy: (a) ability to withstand pressure of external events; (b) capacity to tolerate uncertainty, deprivation and frustration; (c) absence of blindly compulsive activity; (d) freedom from symptoms; (e) increased productivity; (f) adjustment and pleasure in social and sexual life; (g) good interpersonal relationship and sufficient insight. It is clear that such criteria cannot constitute the objective framework required for scientific evaluation.

Even when agreement can be reached on the aims of treatment, it remains necessary to set up measurable indices of response. These indices should be both valid—in being closely associated with the severity of the disease in question—and discriminating, in accurately reflecting responses to treatment. The indices should also be repeatable, preferably simple, and as objective as possible. As a rule the physical correlates of an illness conform to such requirements more readily than do social or psychological criteria. In the present state of knowledge, however, there are relatively few physical correlates of psychiatric disorder. With depression, for example, Eugen Bleuler's statement that "the affect is the index of the whole picture" still remains substantially true, enforcing the use of necessarily subjective criteria in evaluating treatment.

Although the difficulty in standardizing subjective responses to psychiatric treatment led to their virtual neglect for many years, the patent importance of such responses for clinical research in psychiatry has recently led to a quickening of interest in their measurement and assessment. Much work in this sphere has been focused on the construction of rating scales (Wittenborn 1964, see also Chapter 12). Such scales must contain items of behavior that are appropriate to the investigation being undertaken. These items should be pretested to ensure that:(1) they are clearly comprehensive, (2) they apply to the relevant sample of patients, and (3) that they form a progressive continuum. If possible, a scale should also be empirically validated before it is adopted for use in clinical trials. Elaborate but essentially meaningless statistical procedures cannot be justified for their own sake.

THE ANALYSIS OF RESULTS

Since the therapeutic trial is designed to refine clinical experience in quantifiable terms, the statistician, in order to make a maximal contribution, must be involved at every stage of the trial. He should be able to help decide whether the standard comparison of groups is to be preferred to some other design, such as the self-controlled, self-recorded trial (Hogben and Sim 1953), or to the newer sequential techniques (Sainsbury and Lucas 1959). The statistician should also be consulted on dosage schedules as well as on the more specialized problems of recording of data and analysis of results. Only when the statistician is familiar with the material from the outset can full benefit be obtained from his advice, which will be directed towards obtaining clear-cut results whenever possible. Furthermore, in the context of the clinical trial, Bradford Hill has pointed out that the term "not statistically significant" should be equated with the verdict of "non-proven" rather than that of "not guilty."

SPECIFIC AND NONSPECIFIC EFFECTS OF TREATMENT

It is evident that—in theory at least—the modern clinical trial can be modified to evaluate any form of treatment for any form of illness. If in practice it has proved most effective when the physical components of the treatment and illness have been salient, this is principally because these dimensions can be measured most accurately. At present, however, the majority of physical treatments in psychiatry are empirical and precise indications for their use are lacking; thus, clinical trials often yield no more than a broad area of information whose relevance to individual patients may be remote.

When physical treatment in psychiatry rests on a rational basis, however, the clinical trial can be employed to tackle questions of a different order. Speculation about the mode of action of psychotropic drugs, for example, has led to a number of hypotheses, among the most prominent of which involve the role of monoamine oxidase inhibition in the treatment of depression. Thus as discussed in chapter 5, the substance iproniazid (isopropylisonicotinic acid hydrazide) has, following the observation of its euphoriant action in the treatment of tuberculosis, been used in the treatment of depressive states. It is known to exercise an inhibiting effect on monoamine oxidase, the enzyme largely responsible for inactivating 5-hydroxytryptamine, as well as on a proportion of naturally occurring catecholamines. One clinical trial carried out with this drug was designed to learn not merely whether iproniazid benefited depressed patients, but also whether those patients who responded to it could be distinguished clinically and biochemically from nonresponders (by estimations of their urinary 5-hydroxyindoleactic acid output). Still more precisely, the trial was designed to show whether the positive responders exhibited any evidence to suggest that their responses were related to changes in their brain concentrations of 5-HT or of catecholamines (Pare and Sandler 1959). Another example of a biologically oriented experiment carried out within the framework of a clinical trial was designed to test the hypothesis that depressed patients who respond to desmethylimipramine metabolize this drug more slowly than those who do not respond to it, thereby giving the drug more time to exert its pharmacodynamic action (Watt et al. 1970).

Such investigations are being rendered more feasible by the development of newer methods for estimating the plasma levels of psychotropic drugs in humans (Curry 1971, Walter 1971). Their potential importance is further enhanced by the possibility that information obtained in such a therapeutic setting may be used to shed light on the physiopathological mechanisms of the psychiatric disease under treatment. This type of biological specificity is also often contrasted with the nonspecific social and psychological factors which can assume so important a role in the outcome of many physical illnesses, especially those that run a chronic course. A number of psychiatric clinical studies have shown how powerful the effects of these nonspecific or non-drug factors are in the treatment of psychiatric illness, where the interplay between physical and psychosocial factors is more complex and always demands consideration (Shepherd 1961). Partially in consequence of such work, a great deal of evidence has now accumulated about the influence of social factors on the outcome of psychiatric illness. Controlled experiments have indicated the degree of improvement that can be related to environmental change even with chronic schizophrenics (Pasamanick et al. 1967), and it has been demonstrated that the attitudes of such patients are important for the course of their rehabilitation. Only when it is possible to evaluate such supposedly nonspecific therapeutic forces can most current physical methods of treating the major psychoses in

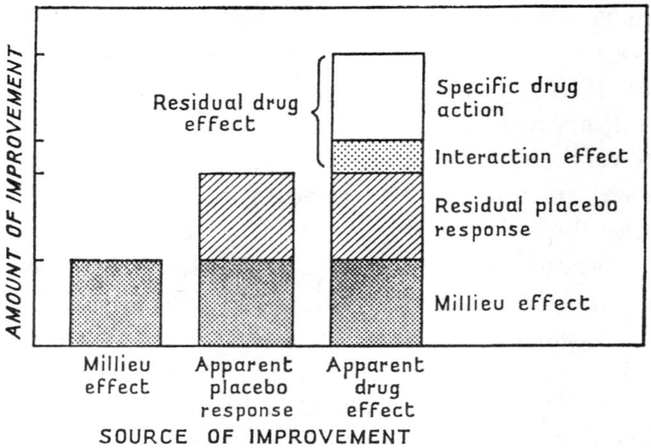

Figure 7-2. Specific and non-specific factors affecting pharmacotherapy in psychiatric institutions. Reprinted with permission from Sainsbury and Kreitman (1975).

institutions be properly assessed, a point which has been well illustrated schematically by Rashkis and Smarr (1958) (Figure 7-2).

In addition to drug therapy, psychological treatments, in one form or another, are also widely used in the treatment of psychiatric illness. Not many workers, however, have been prepared to apply to such treatments the principles governing therapeutic evaluation and, indeed, it has been shown that such an exercise may not be feasible for some forms of psychotherapy (Candy et al. 1972). On the other hand, the introduction of psychological treatments based on learning theory—the so-called behavior therapies—has shown clearly that psychological measures can be subjected to formal evaluation, and this has stimulated their comparison with formal psychotherapy (Gelder et al. 1967).

For their part, while the claims on behalf of formal psychotherapy have been pressed chiefly by enthusiastic but uncritical practitioners and rebutted by equally dogmatic skeptics, very few investigators have so far preferred to study the central problem of such therapy, to which Rosenthal and Frank have drawn attention:

> Improvement under a special form of psychotherapy cannot be taken as evidence for: (a) correctness of the theory on which it is based; or (b) efficacy of the specific technique used, unless improvement can be shown to be greater than or qualitatively different from that produced by the patient's faith in the efficacy of the therapist and his technique—"the placebo effect." This effect may be thought of as a nonspecific form of psychotherapy and it may be quite powerful in that it may produce endogenous changes and relief from stress of considerable duration. [1956]

One of the few investigators who has faced this issue squarely is Leder, who has furnished some evidence suggesting that the psychotherapeutic process be divided into two phases: an initial phase of passive learning when the placebo effect occurs, followed by a phase of specific, active relearning (Leder 1968).

In view of the complexities of this field it is not surprising that much of the most clearsighted work has come from experimentally-minded psychologists, who are more sophisticated than most clinicians in the complexities of experimental design (Edwards and Cronbach 1952). One of the more convincing of these investigations was the treatment of delinquent behavior in the United States Navy by a form of psychotherapy carried out in small closed communities called "living groups," where twenty offenders were placed under the care of three supervisors for six or nine weeks. A consultant psychologist conducted five 90-minute group-therapy sessions weekly, attended by the men and their supervisors. Among the many variables manipulated by the design of this study were the predicted effectiveness of individual supervisory teams, the level of maturity of group members, the duration of supervisor-group relationships, and a variety of interpersonal rating scales. It emerged that the simpler breakdowns of the data failed to do justice to the results; therapeutic success and failure, in terms of subsequent behavior, could be explained only when account was taken of the interaction between predicted supervisory effectiveness and the estimated levels of the subjects' interpersonal maturity.

THE EVALUATION OF MENTAL HEALTH SERVICES

Over the past few years the growing appreciation of the burden of mental disorder on the community has been accompanied by an awareness of the need to introduce and modify both in- and outpatient mental health services. Unfortunately, although a large variety of such measures have been adopted in different societies for different purposes, only a minority of these have been subjected to adequate evaluation. The reasons for this situation are manifold, arising partly from the complexity of the task of evaluation, and partly from the understandable proclivity of health administrators to impose their own values on whatever system of care they adopt. Nonetheless, the need for an objective assessment of such systems is now widely acknowledged, and in the United Kingdom it has been recognized that there is a need to show that "the technique of the controlled trial can be adapted and developed, using sociological and economic as well as clinical measures, so as to play at least a part in the evaluation of complex services" (Matthew 1971).

A number of studies in several areas of the National Health Service are currently under way with this objective. Among the investigations of psychiatric interest there may be mentioned a Scottish case-register study (Baldwin 1971), the Wessex study of mental subnormality (Kushlick 1967), and the community-based program at Chichester (Grad and Sainsbury 1966). The interest of the Department of Health and Social Security in such work should ensure its occupying an important place in the future plans now being formulated.

CONCLUSION

The evaluation of psychiatric treatment should be regarded as no more than a complex variant of a general procedure. Kety (1961) has pointed out that: "Every therapist, be he surgeon, internist, or psycho-therapist, accepts a patient for treatment without knowing all of the individual factors which will determine the final outcome, but on the basis of hypothesis that he can help such patients." While there is still much to learn about the individual determinants of outcome in psychiatric illness, the psychiatrist's therapeutic hypothesis must be put to the test as rigorously as those of other clinicians. Although the task may be a formidable one, the scientific future of treatment in psychiatry depends on the integrity and imagination with which it is tackled.

REFERENCES

Baastrup, P. C., and Schou, M. (1967). Lithium as a prophylactic agent. *Archives of General Psychiatry* 16: 162.

Baldwin, J. A. (1971). *The Mental Hospital in the Psychiatric Service.* London: Oxford University Press.

Blackwell, B. and Shepherd, M. (1967). Early evaluation of psychotropic drugs in man. *Lancet* 2: 819.

Candy, J., Balgour, F. H. G., Cawley, R. H., Hildebrand, H. P., Malan, D. H., Marks, I. M., and Wilson, J. (1972). A feasibility study for a controlled trial of formal psychotherapy. *Psychological Medicine* 2 (4): 545-562.

Curry, S. H. (1971). Chlorpromazine: concentrations in plasma, excretion in urine and duration of effect. *Proceedings of the Royal Society of Medicine* 64: 285.

Doll, W. R. S. (1965). Clinical trials. In *Evaluation of New Drugs in Man,* ed. E. Zaimis, p. 159. Oxford: Pergamon.

Edwards, A. L., and Cronbach, L. J. (1952). Experimental design for research in psychotherapy. *Journal of Clinical Psychology* 8: 51.

Gelder, M. G., Marks, I. M., and Wolff, H. H. (1967). Desensitization and psychotherapy in the treatment of phobic states: a controlled enquiry. *British Journal of Psychiatry* 113: 53.

Grad, J.C., and Sainsbury, P. (1966). Evaluating the community psychiatric service in Chichester: results. *Milbank, Memorial Foundation Quarterly* 44: 246.

Grant, J. D., and Grant, M. Q. (1959). Group dynamics approach to nonconformists in the Navy. *Annals of the American Academy of Political and Social Science* Mar.: 127.

Hill, A B. (1960). In *Controlled Clinical Trials,* ed. A. B. Hill, p. 169. Oxford: Blackwell.

Hill, A. B. (1963). Medical ethics and controlled trials. *British Medical Journal* 1: 1045.

Hogben, L., and Sim, M. (1953). The self-controlled and self-recorded clinical trial for low-grade morbidity. *British Journal of Preventive and Social Medicine* 7: 163.

Kety, S. S. (1961). The heuristic aspects of psychiatry. *American Journal of Psychiatry* 118: 385.

Kushlick, A. (1967). A method of evaluating the effectiveness of a community health service. *Social and Economic Administration* 1 (4): 29.

Leder, S. (1968). Psychotherapy: placebo effect and/or learning? In *The Role of Learning in Psychotherapy,* ed. R. Porter, p. 114. London: Churchill.

Matthew, G. K. (1971). Measuring need and evaluation services. In: *Portfolio for Health,* ed. G. McLachlan, p. 27. London: Oxford University Press.

Medical Research Council (1965). Report by its Clinical Committee: clinical trial of the treatment of depressive illness. *British Medical Journal* 1: 881.

Pare, C. M. B., and Sandler, M. (1959). A clinical and biochemical study of a trial of iproniazid in the treatment of depression. *Journal of Neurology, Neurosurgery, and Psychiatry* 22: 247.

Pasamanick, B., Scarpitti, F. R., and Dinitz, S. (1967). *Schizo-*

phrenics in the Community. New York: Appleton-Century-Crofts.

Pickering, G. W. (1960). In *Controlled Clinical Trials*, ed. A. B. Hill, p. 165. Oxford: Blackwell.

Rashkis, H. A., and Smarr, E. R. (1958). A method for the control and evaluation of sociopsychological factors in pharmacological research. *Psychiatric Research Reports of the American Psychiatric Association* 2: 121.

Rickels, K., Lipman, R.S., Fisher, S., and Park, L.C. (1970). Is a double-blind clinical trial really double-blind? *Psychopharmacologia* 16: 329.

Rosenthal, D., and Frank, J. D. (1956). Psychotherapy and the placebo effect. *Psychological Bulletin* 53: 294.

Sainsbury, P., and Lucas, C. J. (1959). Sequential methods applied to the study of prochlorperazine. *British Medical Journal* 2: 737.

Shepherd, M. (1961). The influence of specific and non-specific factors on the clinical effects of psychotropic drugs. In *Neuropsychopharmacology*, ed. E. Rothlin, p. 183. Amsterdam: Elsevier.

Walter, C. J. S. (1971). Clinical significance of plasma imipramine levels. *Proceedings of the Royal Society of Medicine* 64: 282.

Watt, D. C., Crammer, J. L. and Elkes, A. (1970). *V Conferentia Hungarica pro Therapie et Investigatione in Pharmacologia.* Societas Pharmacologica Hungarica. Budapest, p. 125.

Wittenborn, J. R. (1964). Comments on the selection and use of symptom rating scales for research into pharmacotherapy. In *International Review of Neurobiology*, vol. 7, ed. J. R. Smythies, and D. C. Pfeiffer. New York: Academic Press.

World Health Organization (1967). Research in psychopharmacology. *Technical Report Series.* No. 371.

Zubin, J. (1953). Evaluation of therapeutic outcome in mental disorders. *Journal of Nervous and Mental Disease* 117: 95.

FURTHER READING

Harris, E. L., and Fitzgerald, J. D., eds. (1970). *The Principles and Practice of Clinical Trials.* Edinburgh: Livingstone.

Levine, J., Schiele, B. C., and Bouthilet, L., eds. (1971). *Principles and Problems in Establishing the Efficacy of Psychotropic Agents.* U.S. Public Health Service Publication No. 2138. Washington, D. C.: American College of Neuropsychopharmacology, Inc. and U. S. Department of Health, Education and Welfare.

Shepherd, M., Lader, M. H., and Rodnight, R. (1968). *Clinical Psychopharmacology.* London: English Universities Press.

Chapter 8

Specific and Nonspecific Factors in Psychopharmacology

Scientific dichotomies are often attractively deceptive and in the present context it is necessary to recognize that there are at least two modes of discourse in which the terms "specific" and "non-specific" are loosely employed. The first of these involves the biological concept of specificity. With its roots in the embryological thinking of the late nineteenth century this theme has since been developed, notably in the sphere of molecular biology as well as in genetics (Oppenheimer 1957). Its relevance to the general theory of drug action was clearly outlined by Clark (1937), who distinguished between the selective and the nonspecific effects of drugs on nuclear processes and enzymes.

Laboratory workers with an interest in the biological properties of the psychotropic drugs have commented on the various problems which bear on the identification of specific mechanisms at different levels of function. Thus McIlwain (1957) has suggested that from the biochemical standpoint the mode of action of psychotropic drugs is unlikely to be as sharply specific as that of such substances as the vitamin B group of compounds, in view of their chemical structure and the recent evolutionary status of the system affected by them. In pharmacological experiments Gaddum and Vogt (1956) have demonstrated that a nonspecific antagonism to the central effects of 5-hydroxytryptamine follows the intraventricular injection of compounds as pharmacologically diverse as LSD, morphine, methadone, ergometrine and amphetamine. In the behavioral field Brady (1956) and Sidman (1959) have stressed the need for constructing experiments that take account of the nonspecific emotional responses influencing avoidance reactions; and Cook (1959) has even suggested that a drug effect be regarded as nonspecific if it blocks both the positive conditioned and unconditioned responses, so that specificity of action would be reserved for the suppression of the former response alone.

When we turn to the effects of the psychotropic drugs in humans it is apparent that many of the attempts to examine their specific, or relatively specific, central effects have been offset by difficulties of method and by the notorious variability of human response. Even so, the observations or hypotheses derived from infrahuman studies with these drugs have led frequently to experimental investigations designed to study the degree to which the drugs effects in man can be confined to a particular substance or group of substances. Nowhere does this emerge more clearly than with the Rauwolfia and phenothiazine compounds, whose biological properties have been carefully differentiated but which are still classified together as the "major tranquillizers" and are prescribed interchangeably in clinical practice. Two recent studies with reserpine and chlorpromazine are relevant in this connection.

Following up the suggestions by Burn and Vane that the peripheral pharmacological effects of amphetamine might be related to either noradrenaline release or to a direct 5-HT-like action, Gelder and Vane (1962) administered this drug intravenously to human subjects who had previously received large doses of reserpine or chlorpromazine. During the preliminary control period, blood pressure was taken as the principal index of peripheral response to amphetamine and the psychological reactions, rated by subject and observer, constituted a guide to the central action of the drug. The reserpinized subjects, who had failed to demonstrate the normal, short-lived hypertensive response to an intravenous injection of 10 mg of tyramine—presumably as a result of the depletion of noradrenaline stores—nonetheless responded to amphetamine in the usual way. After receiving chlorpromazine, on the other hand, the same subjects responded to both tyramine and amphetamine with an insignificant rise in blood-pressure. Differences in subjective response were also evident, for following the administration of amphetamine the characteristic malaise exhibited by all of the reserpinized subjects was abruptly terminated and replaced by the mildly euphoric reaction that had been reported in the control period; by contrast, the subjects who had previously received chlorpromazine experienced virtually no affective change.

The second study originated from the hypothesis that the behavioral effects of reserpine in monkeys might be due essentially to the induction of a blockade of incoming sensory stimuli (Weiskrantz 1957). To examine this hypothesis in human subjects, Watt and Crookes studied the response of reserpinized subjects to three groups of psychological tests designed to tap predominantly perceptual, motor, and associational functions, respectively. The subjects were given large uniform doses of reserpine and the tests were administered both when they were receiving the drug and when they were not. The results lent some support to the original hypothesis, since the deficit in the test-performances of reserpinized subjects was demonstrated in the perceptual sphere alone. A repetition of the experiment following the administration of chlorpromazine was then undertaken in order to throw light on the relative specificity of the response to reserpine. In this case the distribution of drug-effects in the various tests was altogether different.

Although on theoretical grounds it can be suggested that an understanding of the specific clinical effects of the psychotropic drugs must depend ultimately on mechanisms of action elucidated in normal human subjects, most of the work with these drugs in humans has in fact so far been directed toward their supposedly therapeutic action. Furthermore, although clinical observations in this field can be directly relevant, as in the seemingly specific response of identical twin schizophrenics to reserpine, discussed by Benaim (1960), the interpretation of clinical reports based on the pharmacological treatment of mental illness is often obscured by the shadow which Henry Maudsley adumbrated sixty years ago. Commenting on the dangers of naive appeal to experience without some knowledge of the character of the experimenter, he pointed out that "in a question of the action of a medical drug he who is least heroic in his use of it, and least confident in his opinion of its powers, will be most likely, in virtue of his mental temperament, to have observed accurately and to have inferred soundly" (Maudsley 1899).

A more fundamental source of error in understanding the specific effects of psychotropic drugs resides in the present ignorance of the physiochemical basis and sequelae of those psychiatric disorders and symptoms that have been most intensively treated with these drugs. It is principally for this reason that the therapeutic action of chlorpromazine in tetanus (Laurence 1957) or of reserpine in hypertension (Dorsett and Woods 1958) can lend itself to a more satisfactory assessment than that of either drug in the functional psychoses. Nonetheless, one of the important byproducts of the current quest for the so-called biochemical lesion in psychotic illnesses has been the submission of the therapeutic response to experimental investigation, since a postulate as well as a proof can be examined by this means. For example, the putative role of monoamine oxidase inhibition in the treatment of depressive states was studied by Dewhurst and Pare (1959) who attempted to relate the clinical responses of depressed patients to the biological activity of one of the monoamine oxidase inhibitors, using a serotonin tolerance test as a direct measure of biochemical function (see Chapter 5). In this way they have demonstrated that clinical status and biochemical activity *in vivo* were largely independent, and thus weakened the case for a specific association between them.

The broad theme of therapeutic specificity leads logically to the second limb of our dichotomy, which was clearly outlined more than twenty years ago in the United States by Cheney and Drewry (1939). Their interest in the pharmacological treatment of mental illness was centered on the then newly introduced insulin treatment of schizophrenia, but they abstained from passing an opinion on its specific therapeutic action; it was left to Ackner and his colleagues (1957) to examine this question directly by employing barbiturate-induced coma to obtain equivalent results. The primary purpose of the American investigators was to demonstrate the need to prove the superiority of the new treatment over the intensive application of accepted methods of good hospital care and management. Calling these general measures "non-specific," they went on to emphasize the importance of establishing the accepted methods' therapeutic possibilities, as a means for setting standards by which any form of supposedly "specific" treatment could be assessed.

At the present time, as insulin units are closing down all over the world, it is imperative to consider the possible relevance of the above canons to the use of the psychotropic drugs, especially in view of the inferences which have already been drawn from the movement of mental hospital populations (Brill and Patton 1959). Perhaps the most far-reaching implications of these canons have concerned the chronic schizophrenics who make up so large and intractable a proportion of psychiatric inpatients in all countries. Unfortunately for the corroboration of therapeutic claims the newer drugs have also served to stimulate dormant staff interest and activities, so that while the resulting changes in mental hospital populations may indicate the previously low level of hospital care, they do not permit an evaluation of the relative roles which specific and nonspecific factors have played in these changes. This point is brought out by the long-term changes which have occurred in one English mental hospital that has been studied in some detail. In the course of the fifteen-year period from 1931 to 1947, it was apparent that patients suffering from the same conditions came to anticipate a shorter stay in hospital, a higher discharge rate, and a lower death rate, all of them indices bespeaking a general improvement in outcome which exceeded the national average (Shepherd 1957). In view of the availability of new forms of physical treatment during this period it was natural to assume that these had been responsible for the amelioration. Closer examination, however, showed that by the end of the fifteen-year period—when physical treatment was freely available—almost 60 percent of newly admitted cases were receiving no form of specific therapy. It then emerged that the latter years had also coincided with the introduction of sweeping administrative reforms which had initiated an all-around improvement in hospital care and the provision of ancillary community services. This policy was undoubtedly responsible in large measure for the improvement in outcome. The same trend in patient flow continued through the early 1950s and the introduction of drug treatment in 1954-55 made little difference either to the overall discharge rate or to the short-term duration of stay, although it did facilitate the routine management of many individual cases. Over the subsequent four years the proportion of schizophrenics admitted to the hospital fell slightly, the numbers remaining virtually unchanged. The resident schizophrenic population remained static, at 53 percent in both 1954 and 1958, while the median duration of stay of these residents actually rose from nine years and eight months in 1954 to ten years in 1957, despite intensive application of drug-therapy; indeed, the proportion of all schizophrenics receiving adequate doses of reserpine and chlorpromazine increased from almost 2 percent to nearly 40 percent in those years.

In this case the pattern of hospital care for schizophrenics that existed before the arrival of psychotropic drugs was not greatly affected by their arrival; most of the therapeutic slack appears to have been taken up over the preceding years. The differences between these findings and the striking changes that have been reported elsewhere may be taken to indicate the therapeutic potential of nonspecific measures. But although statistics make it possible to provide an outline of the clinical effects of nonspecific treatment in terms of quasi-administrative data—and even to frame explanatory hypotheses as Linn (1959) has attempted to do with the material from St. Elizabeth's Hospital—they cannot explore the social and psychological processes through which these effects are mediated. A number of studies of the social setting in which psychiatric treatment is conducted have clearly demonstrated the influence that factors ranging from the physical structure of the ward to the feelings of the nursing staff can bring to bear on even the most malign psychiatric illnesses. Very few social investigators, however, have so far examined the interplay between such factors and the clinical response to psychotropic drugs. One early and instructive example of such work is that of Folkard (1957), a social scientist who employed the techniques of participant observation among chronic psychotics in the wards of an English mental hospital for some months in an attempt to examine the causes and repercussions of aggressive activity. During the course of his study a clinical trial with reserpine was carried out on some of the patients (Wing 1956) with findings that were significant in two respects. Asked to rate the patients' behavior on a formal chart, Folkard recorded no significant changes in either the treated or the control groups, although the doctors and nurses were impressed by the effects of the trial on both. Folkard then analyzed events in terms of aggressive behavior, which he had previously classified by individual characteristics as well as by clinical, social, and interpersonal features, so as to permit a quantitative expression. This procedure enabled him to demonstrate that the sum effect of reserpine treatment could be seen as the quiescence of a relatively small number of patients who had been responsible for provoking others and so initiating disturbances. On the basis of his findings, Folkard was able to argue cogently that attention to particular ward situations, accompanied by the segregation of a few patients, would have been as effective in preventing this "chain" reaction as the physical treatment that had been administered indiscriminately to the whole group.

With changes in the social structure of the mental hospital go psychological adjustments on the part of patients and staff. Perhaps the clearest lead to these intangible factors has come from the study of attitudes, the "neuropsychic states of readiness for mental and physical activity" (Allport 1954), which have often recommended themselves to the social psychologist as an indirect guide to human behavior. An illustrative investigation of these attitudes was carried out at the Medical Research Council Social Psychiatry Unit in London where Wing (1959) studied the rehabilitation of chronic schizophrenics, in hospital for at least two years. He showed that the effects of institutional life can be related to patients' attitudes toward their discharge and their future function rather than to their clinical symptoms or social behavior. It was these secondary attitudes which, in moderately ill schizophrenics, proved to be susceptible to modification by social measures—in this case a period of training in an Industrial Rehabilitation Unit—while the primary handicaps of the disease remained unaffected; furthermore, the improvement was linked closely to the patients' employment status at follow-up.

Within the institution, therefore, it is apparent that the powerful nonspecific factors that bear on the course and outcome of the major psychiatric disorders must be evaluated in assessing the clinical action of psychotropic drugs. Complementary information about the more personal components of drug response has been derived from investigations which have revolved around the nexus between drug effects and the physiological or, most often, the psychological correlates of personality. The meaning and validity of these studies are bound more or less closely to the models of personality on which they are based, and the limitations of such models are attested by the contradictory results that have followed attempts to relate psychological test-batteries, psychodynamic concepts, and factorial dimensions to individual variation in response to low doses of the psychotropic drugs (Brengelmann 1958, Lowell Kelly et al. 1958, Marley and Bartholomew 1959). The same problems have been tackled more directly through the so-called placebo effect, which Wolf has defined appropriately as an effect attributable to "a pill, potion or procedure but not its pharmacodynamic or specific properties" (Wolf 1959). The placebo studies with normal subjects which Joyce (1959) and Knowles and Lucas (1960) conducted in England indicate the importance to response of the conditions of drug administration and the subject's background and relevant experience. These investigators' results find a clinical parallel in the work of Black (1959), who has shown that neurotic outpatients responding to placebo could not be distinguished from nonresponders by formal measures of psychological function, but that the groups were sharply differentiated by their expectations of medical care and by their confidence in doctors. Inasmuch as these findings point to motivation as a significant factor modifying the response to psychotropic drugs, they are in line with the emphasis on incentive, which has been elegantly developed as an operational construct by the Lexington workers in their studies of "post-addicts" (Hill et al. 1957). Their manipulation of this variable to examine the patterns of effect which, they maintain, characterize individual drug responses, represents an approach comprehensive enough to merit wider application.

Even this brief survey shows that an unqualified antithesis between specific and nonspecific factors influencing the clinical effects of psychotropic drugs cannot do justice to the relevant phenomena. Loewi (1952) remarked that the mechanism of drug action depends on some knowledge of what is needed "for the function of the system affected by the drug." If these prerequisites are taken to include psychological and social forces as well as the biological mechanisms to which he was referring, then it becomes the task of neuropsychopharmacology to define these forces and to relate one to the other. In the process many current notions will surely prove to be factitious.

REFERENCES

Ackner, B., Harris, A., and Oldham, A.J. (1957). Insulin treatment of schizophrenia: a controlled study. *Lancet* 2:607.

Allport, G.W. (1954). *The Historical Background of Modern Social Psychology*, vol. 1. Ed. G. Lindzey. Cambridge, Mass.: Addison-Wesley, p. 43

Bartholomew, A.A., and Marley, E. (1959). Susceptibility to methylpentynol: personality and other variables. *Journal of Mental Science* 105:957.

Benaim, S. (1960). The specificity of reserpine in the treatment of schizophrenia in identical twins: a controlled experiment. *Journal of Neurology, Neurosurgery and Psychiatry* 23:170.

Black, A.A. (1959). *Investigation of Placebo Reactors.* Dissertation for the Diploma of Psychological Medicine of the University of London (unpublished).

Brady, J.V. (1956). Assessment of drug effects on emotional behavior. *Science* 123:1033.

Brengelmann, J.C. (1958). D-amphetamine and amytal: 1. effects on memory and expressive movement. *Journal of Mental Science* 104:153.

Brill, H., and Patton, R.E. (1959). Analysis of population reduction in New York State mental hospitals during the first four years of large-scale therapy with psychotropic drugs. *American Journal of Psychiatry* 116:495.

Cheney, C.O., and Drewry, P.H. (1938–1939). Results of nonspecific treatment in dementia praecox. *American Journal of Psychiatry* 95:203.

Clark, A.J. (1937). General pharmacology. In *Handbuchder experimentellen Pharmakologie, Ergänzungswerk,* vol. 4, ed. Heffer, p. 25.

Cook, L. (1959). Comparison of abnormal behavioural states

induced by psychotropic drugs in animals and man (Discussion). In *Neuro-psychopharmacology*, ed. P. Bradley and C. Radouco Thomas, p. 123. Amsterdam: Elsevier.

Dewhurst, W.G., and Pare, C.M.B. (1959). Clinical and biochemical investigation of the action of monoamine oxidase inhibitors in depression. Communication to the *Cambridge Symposium on Depression* (unpublished).

Dorsett, J.D., Jr., Woods, J.W., White, K.L., Smith, H., Jr., and Hill, R. (1958). An evaluation of drug therapy in hypertension. *Journal of Chronic Diseases* 7:287.

Folkard, M.S. (1957). *A Sociological Contribution to the Understanding of Aggression and Its Treatment in a Mental Hospital.*Ph.D. Thesis, University of London.

Gaddum, J.H., and Vogt, M. (1956). Some central actions of 5-hydroxytryptamine and various antagonists. *British Journal of Pharmacology and Chemotherapy* 11:175.

Gelder, M.G., and Vane, J.R. (1962). Interaction of the effects of tyramine, amphetamine, and reserpine in man. *Psychopharmacologia* 3:231.

Hill, H.E., Belleville, R.E., and Wikler, A. (1957). Motivational determinants in modification of behavior by morphine and pentobarbital. *Archives of Neurology and Psychiatry* 77:28.

Joyce, C.R.B. (1959). Consistent differences in individual reactions to drugs and dummies. *British Journal of Pharmacology and Chemotherapy* 14:512.

Knowles, J.B., and Lucas, C.J. (1960). Experimental studies of the placebo response. *Journal of Mental Science* 106:231.

Laurence, D.R. (1957). Some observations on the assessment of drugs in human tetanus. *Clinical Science* 16:443.

Linn, E.L., (1959). Drug therapy, milieu change, and release from a mental hospital. *Archives of Neurology and Psychiatry* 81:785.

Loewi, O. (1952). On the mechanism of drug action. In *Modern Trends in Physiology and Biochemistry*, ed. E.S.G. Barron, p. 405. New York: Academic Press.

Lowell Kelly, E., Miller, J.G., Marquis, D.G., Gerard, R.W., and Uhr, L. (1958). Personality differences and continued meprobamate and prochlorperazine administration. *Archives of Neurology and Psychiatry* 80:241–246.

Maudsley, H. (1899). *The Pathology of Mind.* New York: Appleton, p. 552.

McIlwain, H. (1957). *Chemotherapy and the Central Nervous System.* London: Churchill, p. 303.

Oppenheimer, J.M. (1957). Embryological concepts in the 20th century. In *Survey of Biological Progress,* vol. 3, ed. B. Glass, p. 10. New York: Academic Press.

Shepherd, M. (1957). A study of the major psychoses in an English county. *Maudsley Monograph 3.* London: Chapman and Hall.

Sidman, M. (1959). Behavioral pharmacology. *Psychopharmacologia* 1:1–19.

Watt, D.C., and Crookes, T.G. (1961). The effect of reserpine on perceptual performance. In *Neuropsychopharmacology,* vol. 2, ed. E. Rothlin, p. 410.Amsterdam: Elsevicr.

Weiskrantz, L. (1957). Reserpine and non-behavioral reactivity. In *Psychotropic Drugs,* ed. S. Garattini and V. Ghetti, p. 67. Amsterdam: Elsevier.

Wing, J.K. (1959). *Experimental and Clinical Studies of Rehabilitation in Chronic Schizophrenia.* Ph.D. Thesis, University of London.

Wing, L. (1956). The use of reserpine in chronic psychotic patients: a controlled trial. *Journal of Mental Science* 102:530.

Wolf, S. (1959). The pharmacology of placebos. *Pharmacological Reviews* 2:689.

Chapter 9

Psychosocial Influences on Pharmacotherapy

In comparing the efficacy of pharmacotherapy with that of psychosocial methods of treatment, many investigators give pride of place to drugs—at least for the psychoses—although the arguments on which they base their conclusions are very different. Unfortunately, while their verdict has been endorsed by some authorities, it has also been disputed by others. This therapeutic factionalism is to be expected as long as psychiatrists, while continuing to pay lip service to the concepts of multifactorial etiology and therapy in the sphrere of mental illness, retain individual biases towards either the biological, or towards the social or psychodynamic approaches to treatment. Haefner et al. (1960), for example, have shown that for a group of drug-treated schizophrenics under the care of forty doctors, those physicians who exhibited the most favorable attitudes to pharmacotherapy regarded improvement as greatest. Schulte (1962), on the other hand (as befits a pupil of Hermann Simon), accords to psychotropic drugs no more than a useful supportive role in his occupational and rehabilitative regime, and Lewis (1959) is on record with a substantially similar opinion. Psychotherapy is associated with still another set of values, and the survey of Rose and Esser (1960) in the United States has shown that practicing psychotherapists tend to view drugs as less fundamental and principally useful for symptomatic treatment.

To help reconcile these authoritative but conflicting points of view in a field where opinions outnumber facts, it is obviously imperative to try to answer at least some of the simpler questions by clinical experiments designed *ab initio* to evaluate the relative worth of various forms of treatment. So far there have been disappointingly few studies with this objective. Cowden et al. (1956) treated one group of schizophrenics with chlorpromazine and group psychotherapy and a second with chlorpromazine alone, while taking a third, untreated group as controls. Another trial, which concentrates on the socioenvironmental contribution to treatment, was reported at the Third World Congress of Psychiatry by Grinspoon and Greenblatt (1961). These workers divided 115 chronic schizophrenics into four groups, two of which were treated actively at the Massachusetts Mental Health Center, while the other two remained in a hospital providing only standard custodial care; each pair of groups was then further subdivided, with one subgroup receiving psychotropic drugs, and the others not. The preliminary results, expressed in terms of rating scales and discharge rates, suggested that over the short term, drug treatment was of paramount importance regardless of the environment in which it was used but that with the passage of time the more active therapeutic milieu began to prove its worth.

As far as they go, comparative studies of this type are indispensable, if only to act as brakes on therapeutic zeal.

At present, however, their value is limited by the inadequacy of our diagnostic groupings and our criteria of response. Furthermore, the questions posed by these studies tend to become artificial unless it is recognized that in practice the pharmacotherapy of mental illness is always combined with some form of psychosocial treatment. Unfortunately, the *modus operandi* of modern therapeutic procedures remains so obscure as to handicap efforts to reconcile them—rather than contrast them—within the framework of current therapeutic concepts. The attempt by Ostow and Kline (1959) to link psychodynamic theory with tranquilization through the notion of psychic energy, for example, is more ingenious than convincing. There are therefore immediate practical grounds for paying attention to the work of those investigators concerned primarily with the psychosocial aspects of drug-action.

The effectiveness of a drug is no more than the clinical reflection of one or more of its actions. As it is becoming generally recognized that the effects of drugs on the central nervous sytem represent an interaction between their pharmacodynamic action and the external conditions of the organism to which they are administered, the growing crop of experimental studies on the psychosocial effects of drugs are beginning to assume greater clinical relevance. By comparison, present-day psychological and social forms of treatment are only particular—and probably not very potent—ways of modifying the state of a subject, without having recourse to physical measures.

In the field of human study, the influence of personality on the reaction to centrally acting drugs has long been attested, not only by clinical experience but by controlled observation in the laboratory. The results are well exemplified by the elegant investigation on the effects of small doses of alcohol by Drew et al. (1959), who have shown clearly that the closeness of the relationship between blood alcohol concentration and performance level depends to some extent on defined individual responses to alcohol, as well as on the time that elapses following alcohol ingestion and on the kind of behavior being studied. Another method of inquiry has been through the badly named placebo effect which, as Wendt and Cameron (1961) have pointed out "includes the attitude of the subject towards the experiment, the subject's perception of the experiment, the subject's expectations as affected by the total procedures and his environment both in and out of the laboratory, and the kinds of drugs being used." For the study of environmental factors we are indebted to the social psychologists and the sociologists for indicating not only how the social situation in which an organism is placed at the time of receiving drugs may affect the response to them, but also for indicating what the impact of drug action on such interpersonal concepts as sociability, individual assertiveness and role may be.

So far, as Nowlis (1960) has emphasized, the application of human group models and techniques to the drug field has been limited. Meanwhile, however, workers in the animal field have begun to study socioenvironmental factors as experimental variables in their own right. The careful work of Rosvold et al. (1959) has shown that the effects of so destructive a procedure as neurological lesioning can be analyzed in terms of social behavior indicating that the comparatively less drastic techniques of animal pharmacology might also be expected to facilitate analysis in these terms. Here, perhaps, the best studied phenomena have been those associated with the grouping of animals, beginning with the early work on the toxicity of certain amines by Gunn and Gurd (1940) and later by Chance (1946). The complex interactions between aggregation and other factors such as confinement and temperature have still to be worked out (Höhn and Lasagna 1960) but Lapin (1962) in Leningrad, in studying the puzzling question of why, in spite of their chemical similarities, chlorpromazine and imipramine should have such different effects, has shown by an ingenious set of experiments that the prevention of amphetamine group toxicity can be employed as an index of drug action. Recently Heimstra (1962) has carried the matter further by examining the effects of social stimulation on the behavioral effects of psychotropic drugs, while Swinyard et al. (1961) have provided evidence to suggest that the amphetamine aggregation effect is related to the psychophysiological states of fear or anxiety aroused in individual animals, a theory which may help bridge the gap between this approach and that of the better-known and much larger body of experimental work concentrated on the psychopharmacology of the individual organism (Miller and Barry 1960).

If our understanding of the ways in which psychosocial forces influence the effects of drugs in a clinical setting is to be sharpened, the potential value of experimental studies will have to be explored systematically. There are already problems awaiting investigation. We know at present more about drug-action in relation to the aggregation of rats and mice in their cages than to the grouping of patients on the wards. We know next to nothing about the effects of drugs on interpersonal dynamics. And with a growing tendency for patients to be discharged from hospital on maintenance doses of drugs, clinical observations like those of Richter (1961) on the influence of social circumstances have still to be related to the high- and low-emotional-involvement homes to which Brown et al. (1962) attach importance, and to the findings of Dinitz et al. (1962) on the role performance of discharged patients with the perceived expectations of significant others. For the theme of the psychosocial effects of drugs to be fully developed, however, the clinician and laboratory worker will have to recognize their interdependence.

REFERENCES

Brown, G.W., Monck, E.M., Carstairs, G.M., and Wing, J.K. (1962). Influence of family life on the course of schizophrenic illness. *British Journal of Preventive and Social Medicine* 16:55.

Chance, M.R.A. (1946). Aggregation as a factor influencing the toxicity of sympathomimetic amines in mice. *Journal of Pharmacology* 87:214.

Cowden, R.C., Zak, M., Hayne, J.R., and Finney, R.C. (1956). Chlorpromazine: alone and as an adjunct to group psychotherapy in the treatment of psychiatric patients. *American Journal of Psychiatry* 112:898.

Dinitz, S., Angrist, S., Lefton, M., and Pasamanick, B. (1962). Instrumental role expectations and post-hospital performance of female mental patients. *Social Forces* 3:248.

Drew, G.C., Colquhoun, W.P., and Lang, H.A. (1959). *Effect of Small Doses of Alcohol on a Skill Resembling Driving*. Medical Research Council Memorandum Number 38. London: H.M.S.O.

Grinspoon, L. and Greenblatt, M. (1961). Pharmacotherapy Combined with other Treatment Methods. In the proceedings of the 3rd World Congress of Psychiatry. Toronto: McGill, p. 453.

Gunn, J.A. and Gurd, M.R. (1940). The action of some amines related to adrenaline. Cyclohexylalkylamines. *Journal of Physiology* 97:453.

Haefner, D.P., Sheks, J.M., and Mason, A.S. (1960). Physician's attitude toward chemotherapy as a factor in psychiatric patients' responses to medication. *Journal of Nervous and Mental Disease* 131:64.

Heimstra, N.W. (1962). Social influence on the response to drugs. II. Chlorpromazine and iproniazid. *Psychopharmacologia* 3:72.

Höhn, R. and Lasagna, L. (1960). Effects of aggregation and temperature on amphetamine toxicity in mice. *Psychopharmacologia* 1:210.

Lapin, I.P. (1962). Qualitative and quantitative relationships between Tofranil and chlorpromazine effects on amphetamine group toxicity. *Psychopharmacologia* 3:413.

Lewis, A. (1959). The impact of psychotropic drugs on the structure, function and future of psychiatric services: (a) in the hospitals. In *Neuropsychopharmacology,* vol. 1, ed. P.B. Bradley, P. Deniker, and C. Radouco-Thomas, p. 207. Amsterdam: Elsevier.

Miller, N.E. and Barry, H.I. III. (1960). Motivational effects of drugs: methods which illustrate some general problems. *Psychopharmacologia* 1:169.

Nowlis, V. (1960). Methods for the objective study of drug effects on group functioning. In *Drugs and Behavior,* ed. L. Uhr and J. Miller. New York: Wiley.

Ostow, M., and Kline, N.S. (1959). The psychic action of reserpine and chlorpromazine. In *Psychopharmacology Frontiers,* ed. N.S. Kline, p. 481. Boston: Little, Brown.

Richter, H.E. (1961). Soziale Aspekte der Ambulanten Danestherapie mit Psychopharmaka. *Deutsche Medizinische Wochenschrift* 12:532.

Rose, N., and Esser, M.A. (1960). The impact of recent research developments on private practice. *American Journal of Psychiatry* 117:429.

Rosvold, H.E. (1959). Evaluation of the effects of pharmacological agents on social behaviour. In *Psychopharmacology Problems in Evaluation,* ed. J.O. Cole, and R.W. Gerard, p. 245. Washington, D.C.: National Academy of Sciences-National Research Council.

Schulte, W. (1962). *Klinik der "Anstalts"-Psychiatrie.* Stuttgart: Georg Thieme.

Swinyard, E.A., Clark, L.D., Miyahara, J.T., and Wolf, H.H. (1961). Studies on the mechanism of amphetamine toxicity in aggregated mice. *Journal of Pharmacology* 132:97

Wendt, G.W., and Cameron, J.S. (1961). Chemical studies of behaviour: V. Procedures in drug experimentation with college students. *Journal of Psychology* 51:173

Chapter 10

A Personal View of Clinical Trials

Although doctors disagree as much as most professional men, most practicing physicians seem to accept as their primary function the effective treatment of sick people, preferably on a rational basis, although far too often with empirical measures. It is therefore at first blush surprising to encounter, even in the United Kingdom, the lukewarm opinions often expressed about a peculiarly British contribution to clinical medicine, namely the controlled clinical trial. Perhaps, though, it is necessary to travel abroad to appreciate fully the ambivalence of medical attitudes toward the scientific evaluation of treatment. Commenting on the mixed reception accorded the clinical trial, Walter Modell has turned to social anthropology in suggesting that—

> It is the warm-blooded Latin who resents the suggestion that the scientific approach is essential in the examination of the products of science in man, while it is the cold-blooded Anglo-Saxon who feels that the scientific method

> protects the public against blunders in drug assessment. The United States, still a melting pot, harbors both kinds, the warm-blooded and the cold-blooded, and consequently both attitudes toward the thorough-going scientific trial of drugs in man. Since an attitude toward controlled clinical trials seems more a matter of temperature than logic. . . . perhaps this calls for the antipyretic approach.

I cannot agree. If national achievements indeed reflect national characteristics, I would ascribe the development of the clinical trial in this country less to the British love of the "antipyretic approach" than to a sense of "fair play," a sporting cliche which extends to wider fields. In what other country, for example, could it be said in a national newspaper of a British general retained as chief of staff in the army of a turbulent African country that "His impartiality . . . earned him the respect of a good referee." Again, in his disconcertingly frank account of the process of scientific discovery in *The Double Helix*, James Watson remarks directly on a code of behavior which we in Britain take too much for granted:

> It would have looked very bad if F. had jumped in on a problem that M. had worked over for several years. The matter was even worse because the two . . . knew each other and . . . had frequently met for lunch or dinner to talk about science. It would have been much easier if they had been living in different countries. The contribution of England's coziness . . . plus the English sense of fair play would not allow F. to move in on M.'s problem. In France, where fair play obviously did not exist, these problems would not have arisen. The States also would not have permitted such a situation to develop. One would not expect someone at Berkeley to ignore a first class problem merely because someone at Cal Tech had started first. In England, however, it simply would not look right.

Now in any game the bigger the stakes the more difficult it becomes to ensure fair play. In the therapeutic game there are three parties—the patient, the physician, and the pharmaceutical industry—which for quite different reasons are strongly motivated toward obtaining a positive result. Apart from an understandable desire to get well, the average patient exhibits so pronounced a love of medication as to have moved Sir William Osler to observe that "the desire to take medicine is perhaps the greatest feature which distinguishes man from animals."

On the part of many physicians, as Osler was also well aware, there is a tendency to subscribe to what has been called the touchingly naive assumption of modern therapeutics, namely that there is an answer to every question it poses. On this the late Richard Asher spoke out with his customary frankness when he said:

> If you admit to yourself that the treatment you are giving is frankly inactive, you will inspire little confidence in your patients (unless you happen to be a remarkably gifted actor), and the results of your treatment will be negligible. But if you believe fervently in your treatment, even though controlled tests show that it is useless, your results are much better, your patients are much better and then your income is much better too. I believe this accounts for the remarkable success of some of the less gifted but more credulous members of our profession, and also for the violent dislike of statistics and controlled tests which fashionable and successful doctors commonly display.

Clearly, then, both the patient and the doctor want their treatments to work. What about industry? Despite the statement in a recent textbook that "psychiatric problems are particularly difficult to assess and no doubt because of an honest attempt to relieve humanity of their prevalence, drug houses keep pouring out new agents for their treatment," the verdict of a medical director of one of the larger firms carries more conviction: "Bascially," he said, "our desire is to enable pharmaceuticals to contribute profit to the group."

It is apparent, therefore, that to ensure fair play some rules will be needed, if only to check the combined enthusiasm of the three participants. These rules are provided by the controlled or comparative clinical trial. Understandably, any procedure which can threaten the illusions of the patient, the clinician's belief in his own divine right, and the balance-sheet of the pharmaceutical industry, may be expected to arouse strong feelings. Some of the intrinsic conflicts associated with clinical trials have indeed already been exploited in an effectively dramatic piece of fiction entitled *The Double Blind.*

The arguments in favor of clinical trials are those that go with a desire for medical knowledge and a belief in the progress of clinical science. They can be expected to appeal to all physicians who accept the force of Thomas Huxley's dictum that "Skepticism is the highest of duties; blind faith the one unpardonable sin." In many countries, however, the conditions of medical practice render such an outlook difficult to sustain. The referee's lot is not always easy.

Chapter 11

A Multicentered Clinical Trial

The most elaborate multicentered trial so far conducted in psychiatry was organized by a specially appointed subcommittee of the Medical Research Council of Great Britain. Its purpose was to essay a comparative evaluation of four measures administered to depressed patients in hospital: the measures were electroconvulsive therapy, a tricyclic antidepressant, a monoamine oxidase inhibitor, and a placebo. For inclusion in the trial, the patients, who were of either sex and between 40-and-69 years of age, were required to be suffering from depression as a primary illness with a duration of not more than 18 months. Depression was defined in the following terms: "The primary manifestation and major symptom of the illness to be a persistent alteration of mood (with or without diurnal variation) which exceeds customary sadness, is evident to the examiner, and is accompanied by one or more of the following symptoms: self-depreciation with a morbid sense (or delusional ideas) of guilt; sleep disturbance; hypochondriasis; retardation of thought and action; agitated behavior." Further, the depressed patients should not have received adequate treatment during the previous six months and should not have suffered from serious physical disease. These criteria were established to ensure that the clinical characteristics of the trial population were as homogeneous as possible.

All physicians participating in the trial agreed to treat their patients in hospital for a period of at least four weeks, and thereafter on an outpatient basis unless there were clinical contraindications. During the first month, moreover, the physicians were obliged to accept whichever decision on therapy the organizing team had reached by a process of randomization. In respect to the three tablets—the placebo and the two drugs—the trial was "double-blind." The physicians' foreknowledge of the therapeutic possibilities indirectly imposed another safeguard of homogeneity by influencing the severity of illness. Since each patient stood a one-in-four chance of receiving ECT, a mildly depressed patient would not be subjected to the risk of receiving ECT; nor, by the same token, would a severely depressed patient be exposed to the one-in-four possibility of receiving a placebo. It was, therefore, depression of intermediate severity from which the bulk of these hospitalized patients were suffering.

The attainment of such relative homogeneity, however, was achieved at the cost of easy access to a trial population. For statistical purposes groups of at least 50 patients per treatment were required and three principal difficulties were encountered in seeking these numbers. The first of these was the widespread prescription by general practitioners of antidepressant medication before their patients entered hospital; second, was the reluctance of some physicians to keep their patients in hospital for four weeks; and third was the physicians' understandable wish to protect their patients from either ECT or placebo. The only method of overcoming these obstacles within a reasonable period of time was to ensure the cooperation of a large number of physicians. Eventually, 55 physicians from 30 hospitals widely separated in space were recruited; even so, it was nearly two years before the requisite number of cases was obtained.

The relatively large number of physicians bestowed another advantage on the investigation, namely the possibility of spreading the heavy burden of data collected about each case. The follow-up period was six months from the date of admission—a period judged long enough to assess not only the immediate response to treatment but also the maintenance of that response. The same psychiatrist was asked to assess the patient's condition on specially designed forms at the time of admission to the trial, at weekly intervals during the first four weeks in hospital, just before discharge, and at the end of the second, third and sixth months. Ratings were made on an overall assessment of severity and on each of fifteen specified symptoms. Over the six-month period a predetermined sequence of treatment, to which I will later refer, was laid down.

The importance of ensuring an adequate follow-up made it necessary to pay particular attention to practical details. The maintenance of so elaborate an organization demanded the establishment of a central office staffed by personnel familiar with the administrative aspects of medical statistics. To ensure the collection of sufficient data of adequate quality it was necessary to appoint in addition a full-time secretary and a social worker and to have one highly qualified physician devote at least one day a week to the trial for a period of more than two years. In a study of this type the morale of participating physicians comes to be a cardinal factor if interest is to be sustained and the quality of recording maintained over several months. The small number of patients allocated to each physician—no more than three or four as a maximum—ensured that any potential disaffection could not be attributed to overwork; the danger was rather that the doctors felt themselves to be on the periphery of a large mechanical operation and in consequence to be of little account. Occasional group meetings seemed quite insufficient to counteract this feeling of impersonality. Nor would money ensure the professional interest necessary for full cooperation. The only way to secure this interest was through personal, individual, regular contact by the supervising physician and the social worker; from these contacts it was possible to establish that some physicians preferred to receive reminders by post or telephone, others through diary-cards or their equivalent. Another vital function of the social worker was to trace patients who failed to attend for follow-up and either persuade them to attend the outpatient clinic or obtain the necessary information from them herself. As an index of the success of this procedure, satisfactory information was obtained on 250 of the 269 patients originally admitted to the trial, 222 of these from the physician's reports, 28 from the social worker's. Three patients died during the follow-up period and only 16 were lost.

Separate mention may be made of one issue central to an investigation of this type, namely the ethical responsibility of all participating physicians toward their patients. Inasmuch as they were asked to expose patients to a randomly allocated choice and sequence of treatment, and to withhold supplementary treatments, these doctors were accepting an externally imposed pattern of therapy. It was made clear that at any time they were free to take independent action in the patient's interest. Inevitably, however, this entails further depletions which must be anticipated by aiming at a larger number of patients than is strictly necessary.

So much for some major points of method relating to the design and prosecution of this investigation. They lead up to the problem of evaluation of treatment. The central problem of evaluation is the construction of an index of the condition under study which reflects its progress in objective terms which are, perferably, easy to measure. Unfortunately, despite the many biological and psychological studies of depression which have accumulated over the past fifty years we are still unable to refute Bleuler's assertion, made in 1910, that "the affect is the index of the whole picture." Advances in our knowledge of physiopathology and pathology have not proved firm enough for us to substitute more precise indices; nor, in the opinion of many workers, has refined clinical observation, with its emphasis on syndromes and symptom patterns, added much more, even when elaborated by the statistical techniques which are now, rather late and perhaps surprisingly, finding favor among some psychiatrists—a generation after their limitations have been exposed by our colleagues in psychology. In a planned experiment, however, it is possible to take advantage of the opportunities provided by controlled clinical behavior to establish and monitor a number of indices at different phases of the experiment. These are conveniently subdivided into *short-term indices,* covering the first four weeks, and *long-term indices,* covering the entire six months. The detailed statistics underlying the following summary can be found in the published report of the investigation (Medical Research Council 1965).

SHORT-TERM INDICES

1.The first of these arose from the random allocation of treatments to be maintained for a minimum period of four weeks. This furnished an early opportunity to examine the short-term effect of these procedures since in conditions under study the discontinuation of any treatment could reasonably be taken to indicate dissatisfaction with its value by the physician concerned. As it happened, sixteen of the patients originally on tablets had their treatments changed to ECT before the expiration of the fourth week; only two of these, however, had been receiving imipramine while the remainder were equally distributed between patients on phenelzine and those on placebo. In no instance, on the other hand, was ECT changed to tablets during this time. Here, then, is a first pointer to the relative merits of the four treatments.

2. Direct support to the above view was furnished by the weekly ratings of patients during the first four weeks. These ratings demonstrated clearly that the administration of imipramine was associated with a greater improvement then seen with either phenelzine or placebo. The response to ECT, however, was still more favorable. This finding, furthermore, was independent of the severity of depression and extended to a wide range of symptoms.

3. A third short-term index of evaluation was related to the choice placed before the responsible physician at the end of the fourth week according to the patient's response to initial treatment. The trial conditions specified that if, in the physicians' opinion, a patient were by then well enough he or she should continue treatment on the original tablet according to a prearranged schedule. To patients needing further hospital treatment the physicians agreed to give ECT to drug-treated patients and either of the two active preparations, randomly allocated, to those who had failed to respond to ECT. These circumstances made it possible to attach some significance to the decisions reached at the end of the fourth week, at which time it seemed reasonable to infer

that maintenance of the original treatment would betoken satisfaction with clinical response, just as a change in therapy would suggest a failure to respond. Such changes were deemed necessary in more than half the patients originally on phenelzine or placebo but in only one-third of the patients who had received imipramine or ECT. This distinction was also confirmed by the differences in ratings, after one month, between patients who did and did not then receive other therapy.

LONG-TERM EVALUATION

Interesting as they are in themselves, short-term measures cannot be taken as adequate without regard to evaluation over a longer period. This is true since the course of so many depressive illnesses must be measured in longer terms than four weeks. It was therefore necessary to consider two long-term indices to take into account the natural history of these conditions.

1. The first of the two long-term indices simply represents an extension of the doctors' early decisions about therapy. If, it was argued, the physicians were so satisfied with one of the initial treatments that they employed no other over the entire six-month period, an adequate response could be assumed. By this criterion ECT and imipramine proved superior to the other two tablets over the longer period. A finding of some significance in this context was the maintenance of placebo-therapy in one third of cases.

2. The second long-term index was constructed around the complicated question of discharge from the hospital. The design of the trial rendered this action accessible to analysis. In practice it was found that, while a majority of physicians kept to the prescribed sequence of treatment for eight weeks, it was neither clinically nor ethically feasible to hold them to any detailed therapeutic

pattern after the second month. On the other hand, all participating physicians were committed to discharging their patients from the hospital, either at the end of the four-week period or as soon thereafter as possible, a course of action which accorded well with clinical practice. Here, then, was another piece of clinical behavior which could be taken as a criterion of improvement. Furthermore, discharge is important as a pointer to the speed of therapeutic action, a most important consideration in view of the distressing nature of depression and the shadow of suicide. While the decision to discharge a patient does not, of course, depend solely on the patient's mental state, there was no reason to assume that adventitious factors did not operate equally throughout the four treatment groups. Discharge from the hospital was therefore taken as an index of substantial clinical improvement. However, it was also deemed advisable to refine this index by employing the concept of *final discharge,* defined as discharge without readmission during the following six months and without the administration of ECT on an outpatient basis during this period.

Of the 98 patients remaining on their original treatment, 71 achieved their final discharge by the eighth week, a further testimony to the meaning of maintained therapy. While the administration of ECT was associated with a clear-cut advantage for the first two months, by the end of the twelth week, the final discharge rate of all four initial groups had become equalized. This is understandable since the physicians had been free to employ any form of treatment to help unresponsive patients. Among those patients who had received only the initial treatment until this time, however, ECT and imipramine were both associated with a significantly better response than either the placebo or the MAO inhibitor. It is also noteworthy that, despite the differential effects of the three tablets, ECT was required to produce a favorable response after the administration of all three, in almost the same proportions.

What, then, can we conclude from this study? First, in terms of short- and long-term indices the administration of ECT and imipramine was initially associated with an increased frequency of response beyond that associated with the placebo. Phenelzine, in contrast, demonstrated no advantage over the placebo. Second, ECT acted more quickly than imipramine. Third, about one sixth of the patients needed ECT regardless of what drugs they received. Fourth, about one-third of the patients receiving the placebo alone did well on it. Fifth, about one-sixth of the patients fared poorly whichever treatment they received. The implications of these findings are assuredly of some importance for all workers in this complex field.

REFERENCE

Medical Research Council (1965). Report by its clinical committee: clinical trial of the treatment of depressive illness. *British Medical Journal* 1: 881-886.

Chapter 12

The Treatment of Depressive Illness and its Assessment

QUANTITATIVE METHODS OF ASSESSMENT

Quantitive methods play a major part in the evaluation of new therapeutic substances. Much of the pioneer work in this field dates from 1931 when the Medical Research Council of Great Britain set up its Therapeutic Trials Committee. This soon established the medical statistician as a member of the evaluation team, alongside the clinician and pharmacologist (Green 1954). In the clinical assessment of a new drug it is now generally agreed that after the basic pharmacological data have been acquired from preliminary animal experiments and pilot trials on human subjects, the information gathered should be applied to the measurement of specified reactions against different doses of the drug. It is also necessary to establish the relationship of these reactions to the outcome of the disorder, a step which entails some knowledge of the course of the disorder either without treatment or with some other form of treatment. It is then possible to proceed to the organization of the therapeutic trial which, in its classical form, is designed to compare the effects of treatment in two or more groups, to each of which have been randomly allocated patients differing only in respect to the treatment administered. The criteria of response to treatment should be as unambiguous as possible. A member of the Statistical Research Unit of the Medical Research Council has pointed out that "whenever possible objective and preferably measured assessment of the progress of patients should be used. It is, however, probable that this will have to be supplemented by subjective assessment" (Sutherland 1958). Unfortunately, the difficulty in standardizing subjective responses however, has, until recently, led to their virtual neglect in this field.

The controlled therapeutic trial is not, of course, necessary for the assessment of all remedies. Such trials can be dispensed with if a previously fatal condition can clearly be treated successfully—as in the treatment of tuberculosis meningitis by streptomycin—or when a new remedy is clearly superior to its predecessors—as in the treatment of scrub typhus by chloramphenicol. Furthermore, ethical considerations may limit the possibilities of a clinical trial in some instances. This is especially true if there is evidence that irreversible harm might be prevented by the administration of an existing treatment. Nonetheless, insofar as it has introduced the well-tried principles of prophylactic evaluation into experimental therapeutics, the modern clinical trial enforces a healthy respect for the scientific method in a field where this has not always been prominent. It is important to remember at the same time that the comparative clinical trial is essentially an epidemiological procedure. As such, it reflects the outlook of the statistician, who inevitably tends to think less as a physician than as a metaphysician, specializing therefore in describing the types of proof appropriate to various types of assertion. The commonest form for making such assertions about the therapeutic value of psychotropic drugs has led to clinical trials designed to answer such questions as whether patients suffering from condition X are more likely to benefit from treatment A than from treatment B (which may be a placebo). Whether such a question can be answered with confidence depends in large measure on the precision with which it is possible to define the clinical condition, as well as to specify the criteria of benefit. On both these counts depressive states raise particular problems.

The definition and scope of the illness to be treated is of prime importance for the construction of representative patient samples. Unfortunately, no classification of affective conditions in clinical terms can yet be more than provisional, and recent work purporting to distinguish depressive syndromes by means of the mathematical analysis of symptom-clusters has but largely confirmed the judgment of clinical experience.Based on the most reliable figures we possess, namely the large-scale national statistics of hospital admissions, there is a wide variation in the estimated frequency of these depressive illnesses. In England and Wales the manic-depressive psychoses, most of them in the form of depressive states, make up the largest diagnostic group among cases admitted to mental hospitals. By contrast, in the United States and the Scandinavian countries—where hospital statistics are also carefully compiled—the manic-depressive psychoses and involutional melancholia combine to form a relatively small proportion of cases, while schizophrenia is the condition diagnosed most frequently. This discrepancy cannot be explained wholly by true differences of prevalence. Idiosyncratic classification is partly responsible: the "psychogenic psychoses" of the

Scandinavian authors, for example, include a number of illnesses which would be regarded as depressive elsewhere. The traditions of diagnostic practice itself can also affect the relative estimates of the two major functional psychoses; thus American psychiatrists appear to be guided more than we in Great Britain by Nolan Lewis's dictum (1954) that "the diagnosis of manic-depressive psychoses can be made only by the elimination of schizophrenia." Beyond this, the various prevalence rates of depressive illness, provided by responsible workers, indicate the need to consider the degree of disability leading to inclusion in the diagnostic category. Thus, Fremming's surprisingly high figures from the island of Bornholm must be interpreted in the light of his painstaking survey methods and the finding that 40 percent of his cases had not been under psychiatric care (Fremming 1951). Our experience in Great Britain has shown that patients suffering from the milder forms of depressive illness have tended to enter mental hospitals in increasing numbers as provision for their treatment on a voluntary basis has been extended (Walker 1958), and that many other cases of depressive illness require outpatient services for their detection.

It is apparent that if disregarded this clinical diversity will undermine the structure of a comparative trial, which depends on commensurate severity of illness in both the treated and control groups. Furthermore, the groups must be homogeneous with respect to outcome if the comparison is to be valid. Here the tendency of depressive illnesses to run a self-limiting and often recurrent course renders prognosis difficult in even the better-defined syndromes. It is also necessary to take cognizance of the appreciable mortality rate carried by the major depressive psychoses. Norris (1959), for example, has shown that the crude death rates for men and women suffering from depressive conditions are respectively nine and six times the corresponding death rates for persons of 16 years or older in the general population.

When reasonably homogeneous groups can be constructed, the indices of response have to be defined. The clinical pharmacologist who employs quantitative methods to compare therapeutic substances may proceed by employing one of three methods (Gaddum 1954). These are: (1) the direct assay, in which measurement is made of that dose just necessary to produce an effect; (2) the measured response of a dependent variable; and (3) the assay by quantal (all or none) responses, which are not measured but recorded as being present or absent. With these three techniques, it is possible to study dose-response data according to the conditions of the experiment. Unfortunately, the disturbances of function that accompany depressive states are insufficiently constant or sensitive to be employed in the way in which, for example, blood pressure can be used in the evaluation of hypotensive agents. This is true even for those physiological indices, like weight and certain autonomic responses, as well as such psychological concomitants as altered psychomotor reactions, that are related intimately enough to some depressive illnesses to bear on their prognosis. Sixty-five years ago Eugen Bleuler (1912) commented of melancholia that "the affect is the index of the whole picture," and most of the reported physical and psychological changes seen in depression must still be regarded as epiphenomena. For this reason, in our present state of knowledge the outcome of depressive illnesses and their response to treatment have still to be expressed acceptably in the holistic terms of clinical and social morbidity.

Ethical considerations demand that patients included in a clinical trial should not be deprived of the best available therapy. In many of the milder depressive illnesses this often comprises some non-specific form of pharmacological treatment or some form of psychotherapy. For a large proportion of the more severe illnesses, however, electric shock therapy is available and cannot be lightly withheld in favor of the experimental testing of a new compound. In all comparisons it is necessary to bear in mind that ECT, which despite much work and speculation remains an empirical procedure, carries a negligible mortality and that there are relatively few physical contraindications to its application when administered correctly. It is, nevertheless, a traumatic procedure which many patients and physicians find distasteful.

Convulsive therapy has not been subjected to a formal therapeutic trial; most attempts at its evaluation have been based on a comparison between the outcomes of illnesses treated by ECT in the hospital and the outcomes of the same illnesses recorded by hospital controls in the pre-shock era (Ödegaard 1954). These studies have shown that convulsive treatment reduces hospital mortality rates among patients with depressive illnesses (Slater 1951) and that it also reduces the time which many of these patients spend in hospital (Mayer-Gross 1951). Only twenty years ago mental hospitals could demonstrate the spectacle of whole wards containing "chronic melancholics, who had been in the hospital for two to over twenty years. They had lost the sharp edge of their depression but were anergic, almost inaccessible to stimulation and preoccupied with delusions of unworthiness, hopelessness and physical illness which gravely incapacitated them. Some spontaneously remitted, but there were always others to take their place" (Cook 1958). This corner of mental hospital life has largely disappeared following the introduction of ECT. Several workers have since used the duration of stay in hospital as a useful indication of the severity of illness. They have shown that ECT can cut short and fragment many depressive reactions, particularly in the involutional period, but that it does not influence the disease cycle of the individual patient who exhibits periodic attacks of depression. Furthermore, ECT is without detectable benefit in a proportion of cases from which, on clinical grounds, favorable response would be anticipated.

At present, there is no pharmacological substance whose efficacy can match that of ECT in the treatment of major depressive illnesses. Many drugs have been tried and found wanting—amphetamine and its congeners, the barbiturates, endocrine preparations, dinitrile succinate, methylphenidate and iproniazid, to mention only a few—but it is now more necessary than ever to specify our expectations of any effectice substances which may become available. Even though a drug were to be introduced on an empirical basis it would, of course, be necessary to ensure that it was without serious side effects and that it was of low toxicity; this lesson has been very recently exemplified by iproniazid. If a new substance were no more effective than ECT, it would probably find favor anyhow, because of the advantages attached to its mode of administration, especially if this were by the oral route. In some instances these advantages might prove decisive even if dry therapy were in some measure inferior to ECT, for example in its speed of action. To establish its superiority over electroconvulsive treatment on clinical grounds a new drug might be responsible for one or a combination of the following effects: (1) it might reduce or abolish the mortality rate associated with depressive illnesses treated with ECT; (2) it might curtail the duration of the treated illness, or mitigate still further the social disability associated with the illness; (3) it might prevent subsequent attacks of the illness; (4) it might prove to be efficacious in cases which had failed to respond to electoconvulsive treatment.

It is important to specify which of these features is being singled out in a comparative trial of a drug with ECT. By way of example there may be cited an experiment which we considered with a drug reputed some years ago to be of value in the treatment of depressive states in the senium. Such illnesses display several clinical and biological features in common, and we attempted to secure further uniformity by choosing only patients admitted to our own geriatric unit. The patients, most of whom were in their seventh decade and suffering from affective illnesses uncomplicated by organic features, enjoyed in general a good prognosis, with an average period of stay in hosptial of three months. It had always been the practice of our unit to assess patients for a period of time in hospital before the commencement of active treatment. Advantage was taken of this pretreatment interval to introduce a double-blind procedure with drug and placebo over a period of about four weeks during which ECT was withheld. During this time blood pressure and weight were recorded, biweekly ratings of behavior were made by doctors and nurses, side effects were noted, and different dose schedules of drug were prescribed. Each case was reviewed at the end of this initial period, when the need for further treatment was considered, and ECT was then administered if it was considered necessary. The relevant results of this experiment are summarized in the table below.

Although they have not been included in the table, the dosages of drug administration were equally distributed among all groups. From these figures it is apparent, first, that most patients required ECT after the trial period on the drug; second, that a successful outcome was largely associated with the administration of ECT; and third, that there was no significant difference between the outcome of drug-treated and placebo-treated groups, whether electroconvulsive treatment was administered

Table 12-1
Comparative Trial of a Drug and ECT

Outcome 3 months after admission	*Patients given ECT*		*Patients not given ECT*	
	After Placebo	After Drug	After Placebo	After Drug
Discharged well	8	11	1	1
Discharged with symptoms	10	5	5	7
Remaining in hospital	9	12	2	1
Totals	27	28	8	9

Total number of patients = 72

or not. It was therefore possible to conclude that in the treatment of depressive illnesses with these characteristics, the drug used was inferior to electroconvulsive treatment and no more efficacious that the placebo.

Relatively precise answers of this type are possible even with empirical remedies, and refinements of statistical method can sharpen questions about drug efficacy by, for example, indicating, the degree of improvement that would be accepted as clinically worthwhile before the trial commences (Armitage 1954). If, however, there is a rational basis for the introduction of pharmacological treatment, another order of questions becomes possible within the framework of the therapeutic experiment. Thus, in a recent study carried out by Pare and Sandler (1969), iproniazid was administered to a group of depressed patients with the objectives of determining not merely (1) whether the drug was of benefit, but also (2) whether those patients who did respond to it could be differentiated clinically and biochemically (by estimations of urinary 5-hydroxyindoleacetic acid) from those who did not respond and, more specifically (3) whether among the positive responders there was any evidence to suggest that their response was related to changes in their brain concentrations of 5-hydroxytryptamine (5-HT) or of catecholamines. Similarly the recent pharmacological studies that have shed light on the peripheral effects of amphetamine, have suggested further experiments to determine whether these effects are reproduced in the central nervous systems of depressed patients responding to this drug. The theoretical importance of such investigations is considerable since the information they yield in a therapeutic setting may be used to shed light on the mechanism of the disorder under study. This model may receive more attention with the accumulation of relevant information about the properties of substances in current use.

The drug treatment of the less severe depressive illnesses is beset by problems of its own. Sych illnesses include the large groups of loosely termed "neurotic," "reactive," or "exogenous" depressions, often admixed with the clinical manifestation of anxiety. Many of them run a chronic, fluctuating course. In such cases depression may represent a symptom as much as a syndrome and the indices of outcome available for the major depressive illnesses find limited application in their treatment. Only a minority of patients with these lesser depressive illnesses require convulsive therapy. If they do attend hospital they are unlikely to require admission and it seems probable that many of them never come under psychiatric care.

Recent studies of morbidity in general practice under the National Health Service in Great Britain have suggested that depressive illnesses rank high in the psychiatric case-load of the practitioner, and that he treats the majority of mildly depressed patients himself (Watts 1956). From sociomedical inquiries, it also seems probable that other patients suffering from these conditions do not come to medical attention at all but rely; rather on the advice of the chemist or on self-medication. When the disability consists of no more than feelings of discontent, distress or discomfort, even social criteria like the work record may be too crude for purposes of assessment.

It is notoriously difficult to apply the principles of the therapeutic trial to illnesses of this sort. Treatment can be evaluated by a group trial in favorable circumstances (Davies and Shepherd 1955), but there are many practical and theoretical obstacles to this. The dropout rate is high and there is always uncertainty as to whether the patient is taking the drug or not. The diversity within diagnostic categories is considerable and impairs the possibility of generalization from the small numbers of patients that are usually treated for these conditions. Changes in the course of the condition may be linked more with interpersonal and social factors than with the patient's drug treatment. Furthermore, the criteria of response in such trials depend wholly or partly on clinical judgments made by the observer and on ratings of experience or drug preference by the patient, criteria which are inevitably subjective. Finally, the wide individual variation of response to drugs (Von Felsinger et al. 1955) assumes such importance that it may be necessary to employ an experimental design that permits information about individuals to be extracted.

An alternative method of tackling this problem is to concentrate directly on the universe of the individual patient, studying the intra-individual variation. This principle is familiar to physiologists and psychologists (Jellinek 1939, Shapiro 1957). Its application to therapeutics has been advocated by Hogben and Sim (1953) as a means of direct examination of the stimulus-response nexus. What these authors call the self-controlled, self-recorded trial is designed to study the therapeutic response in states of chronic, low-grade morbidity which are not regarded as reversible and where the endpoints of therapy are defined by symptomatic relief rather than by cure. In such studies, the controlled investigation of subjective data in the form of symptoms is a central feature of the experimental design. Symptoms are subdivided for the purpose into those usually associated with disturbances of behavior, so becoming open to observation (e.g. anorexia), and those in which personal experiences predominate rendering the subject's testimony the principal source of data (e.g. referred pain). Our experience suggests that the treatment of less severe chronic depressive states can be investigated in this way. The suitable subject is invited to complete predesigned forms bearing on specified functions and experiences. The forms can be filled in at regular intervals under normal working or domestic conditions. Internal checks are provided for subjective data, and the cooperation of an observer can be enlisted for the verification of functional disturbance. After a period of observation without treatment the effects of modification can be observed, the subject remaining in ignorance of the substances which he receives.

If the initial recordings for such studies are made in hospital the nursing staff will enable an estimate to be made of the reliability of the subject's observations. On discharge the subject's spouse can cooperate in the same way for regular recordings during intervals between psychiatric assessments. Although the intra-individual technique raises several problems in the selection of subjects, the recording of information and the mathematical treatment of summated indices, the data which it provides about natural fluctuations and the continuity of response make it a promising research tool in the study of the elusive, mildly depressive conditions.

It now seems probable that we are soon to be presented with so many new antidepressive compounds that the familiar clinical attitude of laissez-faire empiricism will be increasingly difficult to sustain. The clinician is compelled to hold the balance between the scales of laboratory data on the one hand and stochastic theory on the other. Although his experience and judgment are essential, it will be necessary for him to adopt a more experimental role in the future if he is to cooperate fully with the pharmacologist and the statistician, whose techniques he should understand if full weight is to be given to observations made in the clinical setting. More clinical research is indispensable to progress in the evaluation of drugs for the treatment of depression.

RECENT DEVELOPMENTS

Part I of this survey, which appeared ten years earlier, reviewed the evaluation of pharmacotherapy in the treatment of depression, with special reference to the place of clinical trials. It is now appropriate, therefore, to survey some of the more important developments of the past decade in this field. For convenience the material can be grouped into four general categories: (1) attitudes to clinical trials; (2) the early evaluation of antidepressant medication; (3) the confirmatory evaluation of antidepressant medication; and (4) the prophylaxis of depression.

Attitudes to Clinical Trials

Social psychologists insist that attitudes are precursors to action. As such they warrant consideration in their own right, and it is instructive to recall the opening remarks made by the discussant of my paper 10 years ago on the subject of controlled clinical trials:

> Such studies seem to have undergone a kind of historical waxing and waning. Thus prior to the last decade or two, one seldom heard of them. Once they entered the scene, however, it became fashionable to decry the results that were not "controlled" in this manner. But now the wheel

> has, as it were, turned full circle so that it is fashionable, even perhaps *avant garde,* to heap critical coals of fire upon such an approach. [Sloane 1959]

Clearly, the fire has largely died out since the above statement was made. The changed attitude of the pharmaceutical industry is well attested and many workers in the medical profession have also come to adopt a more critical attitude to therapeutics, possibly associated with the rise of clinical pharmacology as an emerging discipline. Several psychiatrists have questioned both the claims advanced on behalf of antidepressant drugs (Kimbell et al. 1965) and the adequacy of the methods being employed to evaluate them (Leyburn 1967). In this context one of the most instructive reports reviewed all papers concerned with the evaluation of antidepressant medication published over a five-year period in 17 American, British, and Canadian journals (Wechsler et al. 1965). The authors identified seventy-nine separate studies, of which thirty had been conducted without controls, twenty-two with placebo controls, and twenty-seven with active drug controls.

A more detailed analysis of the above papers made it possible to draw several conclusions of general interest. First, there was considerable variability in the reports on any one medication, and assessments of efficacy ranged from nil to one hundred per cent. Second, the type of research design was related to reported outcome: in general, studies in which placebos were employed yielded the lowest estimates of efficacy. Third, in studies where placebo was used, an improvement on the drug tended to be associated with improvement on the placebo. Fourth, the administration of electroconvulsive therapy was more effective than any form of medication. It is surely important to emphasize these findings as a background to any individual study in clinical drug evaluation.

The Early Evaluation of Antidepressant Medication

Reviewing research in psychopharmacology, a World Health Organization scientific group has subdivided the stages of clinical drug evaluation into three phases (World Health Organization 1967). Phase I concentrates on a determination of the effective drug range, adverse effects, and possible toxic properties of a new drug; such work depends on experience and careful clinical observation, and is usually carried out on groups of from five to twn patients as a therapeutic experiment without controls. Phase II trials are concerned with the therapeutic range and effectiveness of the drugs which are studied; these trials may or may not be controlled but should be conducted with larger groups, of the order of from ten to thirty, by some investigator in the WHO report apotheosized as "a perceptive observer, able to use imagination and follow clinical 'hunches.'" Together, the first and second phases of clinical trials constitute the stage of early evaluation, in which it is possible to make observations that can later be validated by the more strictly controlled techniques of phase III.

In the sphere of antidepressant medication the stage of early evaluation has been most neglected. This is partly due to the difficulties posed by the use of animal behavior for the study of affective phenomena in humans. The logic of the pharmacologist may, of course, dismiss this obstacle as chimaerical, as in the following example:

> How does one study the antidepressive action of a sedative? Obviously, normal animals cannot be used; we must somehow set up a model depression in animals. But depression does not have the same meaning to a physiologist as it does to a psychiatrist, and I did not wish to become entangled in semantic difficulties. I asked a psychiatrist friend to describe to me the symptoms of endogenous depression in a subject who had only recently acquired the disease. It

> seemed to me that I was listening to a description of the action of reserpine—even to its parasympathetic effects. We decided therefore that our model depression would be the syndrome of effects elicited by reserpine or reserpine-like compounds. [Brodie 1965]

However satisfying such a simplified view may be to its originators, it is not supported by experimental or clinical facts; there is still no adequate substitute for the human subject when depression is to be investigated or treated. Unfortunately, however, the first administration of a new antidepressant drug to humans all too often exemplifies what has justifiably been termed a "leap in the dark."

It was with this problem in mind, and with an awareness of the dearth of investigations designed to tackle it, that we attempted to explore some of the practical and theoretical aspects of early evaluation with a new antidepressant compound at the Institute of Psychiatry. Our objectives were to examine whether the oral administration of the drug to depressed inpatients was effective and, simultaneously, to assess both the drug's side effects and its action on hematological, hepatic, renal and cardiovascular function. Inasmuch as we were concerned with trying to devise a method for testing new antidepressants on a restricted number of patients before release in large-scale trials, we were, in effect, combining phases I and II in a single operation.

This work has been fully reported (Blackwell and Shepherd 1967). It demonstrates conclusively how many practical and administrative hurdles lie in the path of the investigator who would follow this track. Here I would mention only one such obstacle, the problem of obtaining suitable patients. Thus, although we were working in a large and relatively well-staffed institution with access to many patients, only six of the fifty depressed subjects who met the criteria for inclusion in the study completed the trial. The reasons for the heavy loss of patients included refusal of consent by the patient, relative, or consultant; the existence of a complicating physical condition; rapid remission or self-discharge from hospital; such worsening of illness as to require electroconvulsive treatment; and a history of previous treatment with a similar drug. It is evident that despite the mutual interest of the pharmaceutical industry and the medical profession in promoting such research, its organization demands more facilities than are generally acknowledged as necessary. Yet early evaluation remains an outstanding challenge if the flood of new antidepressant drugs is to justify itself.

The Confirmatory Evaluation of Antidepressant Medication

In terms of the WHO schema, the phase III controlled trial requires larger groups of patients "so that sensitive statistical tests can be used in evaluating the final results. Phase III trials, therefore, call for carefully conceived and executed experiments and for skillful evaluation of the results." There are, as the report further points out, no fewer than eight possible types of experimental control which may be employed. These are: (1) the comparison of a drug with no treatment, which can be non-blind, single-blind or double-blind; (2) the comparison of one drug with another drug, which again can be non-blind, single-blind or double-blind; and (3) a comparison of a drug with a placebo, which must be either single-blind or double-blind.

The number of controlled trials of antidepressant medications has been steadily increasing over the past decade, but so far the largest and the most impressive is the multicenter investigation organized under the aegis of the Medical Research Council (Medical Research Council 1965). This was designed to compare the efficacy of four treatments (Shepherd 1967a and 1967b). No mention of this study, however, is complete without stressing that it applied only to groups of patients, and not to individuals. All attempts to identify which factors determined individual response to treatment were unsuccessful. The great variation of response within defined groups of depressed patients is clearly of considerable interest in its own right, however, and it has recently been subjected to close analysis from three different points of view, all of which relate to the problems of therapeutic evaluation. These viewpoints are concerned, respectively, with: (1) the classification of depressive disorders; (2) the biological basis of depression; and (3) the social factors bearing on depression.

With regard to the first viewpoint, the importance of an adequate system of classification is apparent. If, as some workers maintain, there are several etiologically distinct types of depressive illness, it would not be surprising to find that our relatively crude clinical criteria fail to distinguish between heterogeneous conditions which respond differentially to the same treatment. Within the limitations of our present knowledge perhaps the most adequate solution to this problem has been proposed by Kendell (1968) on the basis of his analysis of a large series of depressive illnesses with refined statistical methods. His conclusion was "to regard depressions at one pole, the classical endogenous depressions at the other and the majority of patients in between." Furthermore, Kendell goes on to suggest that a mathematically derived index of the depressive condition, along the lines he has developed, can be substituted usefully for clinical concepts. "To say that a patient has a depressive illness with an index score of +4 is more informative than saying that he has a psychotic depression or even that he has a borderline psychotic depression" (Kendell 1968). Here is a line of research which can be adopted profitably in therapeutic experimentation.

As regards the second viewpoint, the biological explanation of the variations in therapeutic response tends to focus on drug metabolism, and this emphasis sometimes leads to direct criticism of the clinical trial in its usual form:

> A biologist sounds a word of warning when he hears that "double-blind" studies are carried out using fixed dosage schedules. The double-blind test involves a sound principle and is meant to separate factors such as variability of the disease process, bias, placebo effects, and so forth. But the use of this test implies that the drug is present in each subject in approximately the same amount in mg/kg. This might be true with highly polar drugs, substances which are not metabolized and disappear from the body at rates that are essentially similar among different individuals. In contrast, drugs that act on the brain, being highly lipid soluble, undergo extensive metabolism at rates that are highly variable from person to person. Thus, the investigator applying the double-blind test in the belief that he is circumventing biological variability, may be substituting a situation in which the biological variability is vastly greater. [Brodie 1965]

The study of individual differences in human drug metabolism is preeminently a task for the clinical pharmacologist. Technical reasons have handicapped its application to the antidepressant field until recently, but the development of new chemical methods has now enabled some workers to demonstrate its relevance. In Stockholm, for example, a sensitive *in vitro* labeling technique has been used to estimate the plasma level of the tricyclic monomethylimipramine antidepressants in humans. Reported data indicate a wide range of individual variation in the plasma levels of desmethylimpiramine and also, incidentally, the interesting observation that disturbing side effects were associated with high plasma levels of desmethylimipramine (Sjoqvist et al. 1968).

With such techniques at hand it also becomes possible to carry out biologically-oriented experiments within the framework of a clinical trial. This has been done by Elkes (1968) who has tested the hypothesis that depressive patients who responde to desmethylimipramine metabolize this drug more slowly than those who do not, thereby giving the drug more time to exert its pharmacodynamic action. It would follow from this hypothesis that unresponsive patients should excrete larger amounts of unchanged drug, there being more of it to excrete, than patients who are responsive to desmethylimipramine. On this assumption Elkes proceeded to employ the general structure and criteria of the Medical Research Council trial of the treatment of depressive illness, in order, first, to eliminate placebo-responders, and, second, to make comparative biochemical observations on those patients who did and did not respond to medication. The rate of metabolism of desmethylimipramine was studied by fluorimetric measurement of the percentage of the daily dose excreted in a twenty-four-hour specimen of urine; in addition, thin-layer chromatography made it possible to display the metabolites of desmethylimipramine and estimate their relative qualities in urine. As it happened, Ekles' results appear to be negative, in that no clear-cut difference emerged between responders, but experiments of this type may confidently be expected to extend the scope of clinical trials of antidepressants drugs as biological methods become more refined.

Concerning the third viewpoint, in addition to clinical and biological variables, account must also be taken of the influence of social factors on the apparent response to pharmacotherapy. Such factors have been shown to bear on discharge from hospital, which is often taken as an index of amelioration (Watt and Buglass 1966). Among such factors marital status is of indisputable importance. Patients with depression are known to enter hospital earlier and stay longer if they are single than if they are married. Further, Angst (1965) has claimed that this relationship remains demonstrable after treatment with antidepressants. We may hope to see this dimension further explored in the evaluation of these drugs in the future.

The Prophylaxis of Depression

The notion of prevention has recently become prominent in the literature on antidepressant medication and is likely to grow in volume. It is implicit in the rationale of maintenance therapy, which is the subject of a current Medical Research Council investigation. Much of the discussion of prevention, however, has so far been focused on lithium carbonate, following the claim that it is "the first drug for which a clear-cut prophylactic action against one of the major psychoses has been demonstrated" (Baastrup and Schou 1967). The fallacies in the logic of this claim have been pointed out elsewhere (Blackwell and Shepherd 1968), but the prospect of preventing depression by chemical means has already proved irresistible in some centers and, in the process, has even resulted in a challenge to the proper use of clinical trials. Thus in Sweden, a double-blind study has been terminated for "ethical" reasons on the following grounds:

> From the start we decided not to include patients with severe affective psychoses—i.e. with very frequent relapse, serious suicidal attempts, and/or long social disablement. These patients were instead assigned to an "open" lithium group, on the grounds that, although Dr. Baastrup and Dr. Schou may not have afforded proof of the prophylactive action of lithium, they have nevertheless provided so much evidence that we felt it unethical to deprive severely ill patients of this chance. Since we formed the impression

> that patients in this open lithium group reacted favorably, and since colleagues from other hospitals reported similar consistent impressions, our unwillingness to deprive patients of lithium increased. From at first excluding only the graver cases, we gradually allowed even milder cases to join the open lithium group, which meant that fewer cases became available for the double-blind study.
>
> Another cause of the failure of the experiment was the publicity that lithium has been given in Sweden, where most psychiatrists believe that its value far outweighs its risks in severe recurrent affective psychoses. Our patients got to know that lithium was considered to have a prophylactic effect, and several of them specifically asked for it. We have known most of our patients for several years; they apply to the clinic when they have a relapse, and thus it was not easy to include them in a double-blind study. In our opinion, it is now too late to make a study in Sweden in which a simultaneous control group is not given lithium. The problem might be less in countries where knowledge of lithium is more limited or the psychological conditions different. [Laurell and Ottosson 1968]

Such a viewpoint, backed up by the asseveration that "observer bias and psychological factors are probably not major sources of error," would seem to bring us back to our point of departure: namely, the importance of attitudes adopted toward clinical trials. Perhaps I may be permitted to conclude this chapter not only by deprecating the attitude exemplified by the foregoing quotation, but by reaffirming what I wrote ten years ago:

> It now seems probable that we are soon to be presented with so many new antidepressive compounds that the familiar clinical attitude of laissez-faire empiricism will be increasingly difficult to sustain. The clinician is compelled to hold the balance between the scales of laboratory data on the one hand and stochastic theory on the other. Though his experience and judgment are essential, it will be neces-

sary for him to adopt a more experimental role in the future if he is to cooperate fully with the pharmacologist and the statistician, whose techniques he should understand if full weight is to be given to observations made in the clinical setting. More clinical research is indispensable to progress in the evaluation of drugs for the treatment of depression.

I would predict that these comments are likely to be still more applicable to the seventies than they have been to the sixties.

REFERENCES

Angst, J. (1965). Erfolg und Misserfolg der psychopharmakologischen Therapie am Beispiel der Depression. *Hippokrates* 36:946.

Armitage, P. (1954). Sequential tests in prophylactic and therapeutic trials. *Quarterly Journal of Medicine* N.S. 23:255.

Baastrup, P.C. and Schou, M. (1967). Lithium as a prophylactic agent. Archives of General Psychiatry 16:162.

Blackwell, B. and Shepherd, M. (1967). Early evaluation of psychotropic drugs in man. *Lancet* 2:819.

Blackwell, B. and Shepherd, M. (1968). Prophylactic lithium: another therapeutic myth? *Lancet* 1:1968.

Bleuler, E. (1910-1912). Affectivity, suggestibility, paranoia. *State Hospital Bulletin*, New York, N.S. 3-4:481-601.

Brodie, B.B. (1965). Some ideas on the mode of action of imipramine-type anti-depressants. In *The Scientific Basis of Drug Therapy in Psychiatry*, ed. J. Marks and C.M.B. Pare, Oxford: Pergamon.

Cook, L.C. (1958). The place of physical treatments in psychiatry. *Journal of Mental Science* 104:933.

Davies, D.L., and Shepherd, M. (1955). Reserpine in the treatment of anxious and depressed patients. *Lancet* 2:117.

Elkes, A. (1968). Mode of action of imipramine. M.D. Thesis. London: University of London.

Fremming, G.H. (1951). The expectation of mental infirmity in a sample of the Danish population. Occasional Papers in Eugenics, Number 7. London: Eugen, Society.

Gaddum, J.H. (1954). Clinical pharmacology. *Proceedings of the Royal Society of Medicine* 47:195.

Green, F.H.K. (1954). The clinical evaluation of remedies. *Lancet* 2:1085.

Hammer, W. and Sjöqvist, F. (1967). Plasma levels of monomethylated tricyclic antidepressants during treatment with imipramine-like compounds. *Life Sciences* 6:1895.

Hogben, L., and Sim, M. (1953). The self-controlled and self-recorded clinical trial for low-grade morbidity. *British Journal of Preventive and Social Medicine* 7:163.

Jellinek, E.M. (1939). The function of biometric methodology in psychiatric research. *American Association for the Advancement of Science*, Publication Number 9, p. 48.

Kendell, R.E. (1968). The problem of classification. In *Recent Developments in Affective Disorders*, ed. A. Coppen and A. Walk, Ashford: p. 15. *British Journal of Psychiatry* Special Publication Number 2. Headley Bros. Ltd.

Kimball, I., Overall, J.E. and Hollister, J.E. (1965). Antidepressant drugs: myth or reality? *Journal of New Drugs* 5:9.

Laurell, B. and Ottosson, J.O. (1968). Prophylactic lithium? *Lancet* 2:1245.

Lewis, N.D.C., and Piotrowski, Z.A. (1954). Clinical diagnosis of manic-depressive psychosis. In *Depression*, ed. P.H. Hoch, and J. Zubin. New York: Grune and Stratton.

Therapie am Beispiel der Depression. *Hippokrates* 36:946.

Lancet 2:1135.

Mayer-Gross, W. (1951). Discussion on the treatment of depression. *Proceedings of the Royal Society of Medicine* 44:961.

Medical Research Council (1965). Report by its Clinical Committee. Clinical trial of the treatment of depressive illness. *British Medical Journal* 1:881.

Norris, V. (1959). *Mental Illness in London: A Statistical Enquiry Into Admission to Mental Hospitals.* Maudsley Monograph Number 6. London: Chapman and Hall.

Ödegaard, O. (1954). Results of treatment in mental hospitals in Norway before and after the introduction of shock treatment. *Mental Hygeine* 38:447.

Pare, C.M.B., and Sandler, M. A trial of iproniazid in the treatment of depression: a clinical and biochemical study. *Journal of Neurology, Neurosurgery and Psychiatry.* In press.

Shapiro, M.B. (1957). Experimental method in the psychological description of the individual psychiatric patient. *International Journal of Social Psychiatry* 3:89.

Shepherd, M. (1967a). Implications of a multi-centred clinical trial of treatments of depressive illness. In *Anti-depressant Drugs*, ed. S. Garattini, and M.N.G. Dukes, p. 332. Amsterdam: Excerpta Medica.

Shepherd, M. (1967a). The method of the multi-centred clinical trial. In *Neuropsychopharmacology*, ed. H. Brill, J.O. Cole, P. Deniker, H. Hippius, and P.B. Bradely, p. 51. Amsterdam: Excerpta Medica.

Sjöqvist, F., Hammer, W., Ideström, C-M, Kind, M., Tuck, D., and Asberg, M. (1968). Plasma level of monomethylated tricyclic antidepressants and side-effects in man. In *Proceedings of the European Society for the Study of Drug Toxicity*, vol. 9, *Toxicity and Side-effects of Psychotropic drugs*, p. 246. Amsterdam: Excerpta Medica.

Slater, E.T.O. (1951). Evaluation of electric convulsion treat—ment compared with conservative methods of treatment in depressive states. *Journal of Mental Science* 97:567.

Sloane, R.B. (1959). Discussion (of paper by M. Shepherd). *Canadian Psychiatric Association Journal* Special Supplement 4:S126.

Sutherland, I. (1958). A symposium on clinical trials. *Pfizer*. Tonbridge: Tonbridge Printers.

von Felsinger, J.M., Lasagna, L. and Beecher, H.K. (1955). Drug-induced mood changes in man. 2. Personality and reactions to drugs. Journal of the American Medical Association 157: 1113.

Walker, L.D. (1958). The pattern of post-war psychiatric practice. Thesis (M.D.). London: University of London.

Watts, C.A.H. (1956). *Neuroses in General Practice*. Edinburgh: Royal College of Physicians Publications Number 6.

Watt, D.C. and Buglass, D. (1966). The effect of clinical and social factors on the discharge of chronic psychiatric patients. *Social Psychiatry* 1:57.

Wechsler, H., Grosser, G.H., and Greensblatt, M. (1965). Research evaluating antidepressant medications on hospitalised mental patients. *Journal of Nervous and Mental Disease* 141:231.

World Health Organization (1967). Research in psychopharmacology. *Technical Report Series,* Number 37. Geneva: World Health Organization.

Chapter 13

Prophylaxis and Antidepressant Medication

Few terms have been applied to psychiatry more hopefully and with less scientific justification than "prevention." It is worth recalling that in the sphere of general medicine this concept is widely employed by public health workers to embrace prevention at three levels: "primary" prevention, aimed at eliminating the cause of disease; "secondary" prevention, aimed at the treatment of established disease; and "tertiary" prevention, aimed at the reduction of disability. The use of medicinal substances is largely concentrated on the second and third of these two levels, and although there has been a growing tendency for the prescription of these medicines to be described as "prophylactic," we should recognize that in this context the word "prophylaxis" can assume several meanings. First, it can imply substitution, the making up of a deficiency. Examples here would include the long-term prescription of a thyroid preparation for hypothyroidism or of vitamin B12 for pernicious anaemia.

Second, it may imply the suppression of an ongoing disorder, as with corticosteroids for a collagen disease or disodium cromoglycate for asthma. Third, it may be employed in relation to the use of one drug as a substitute for another, as in the methadone program for opioid dependence. Fourth, the aim may be the prevention of further attacks of a recurrent disease, as when antibiotics are given to a patient liable to repeated infections.

It is to the fourth of these meanings that it has become customary to apply the concept of "prevention" to manic-depressive disorders. However, unlike the bulk of infectious diseases, both the pathophysiology and the natural history of affective disorders are obscure. Thus the scientific evidence required to establish the supposedly "prophylactic" properties of a drug for such disorders is difficult to establish. The problems of method have been debated most intensively in relation to the putative action of lithium carbonate in preventing further attacks of mania and depression in patients with a history of recurrent manic-depressive illness (Blackwell and Shepherd 1968), an issue which is still *sub judice.* In clinical practice, however, the same type of issue arises much more frequently with regard to the decision to continue with antidepressant medication after the resolution of depressive symptoms, following treatment with one or another of the available preparations. Thus, although there is some evidence favoring the efficacy of tricyclic compounds in the treatment of some forms of depressive illness (Wechsler et al. 1965), there is no satisfactory work designed to assess the need for subsequent medication. In everyday clinical work such medication usually consists of continuation of the same drug, often at a lower dose, for a variable period of time depending largely on the experience and inclination of the individual physician. In the view of those clinicians who believe that the mode of action of the drugs is merely to *suppress* depressive symptoms, without modifying the natural history of an underlying disorder, treatment should be continued until the illness has run its course. In the opinion of others the action of the drugs is more fundamental; for them the primary aim of treatment after symptomatic remission of depression is to *prevent* the recurrence of further episodes, and prophylaxis would therefore become a legitimate objective.

At present, so little is known about the rationale for continuing antidepressant medication after the remission of symptoms that it would seem preferable to use the relatively neutral term *continuation therapy* rather than the widely used but potentially misleading concept of *maintenance therapy.* The latter term has been defined in a current textbook as follows: "A stage in the course of chemotherapy. After the drug has reached its maximal efficacy, the dosage is reduced and sustained at the minimal therapeutic level that will prevent a relapse or exacerbation" (Freedman et al. 1972). Such a definition clearly implies a form of prophylactic action, and because of the frequency and duration of antidepressant medication it is of some socio-economic as well as scientific importance to obtain reliable information on this question. Unfortunately there have been very few controlled studies of continuation therapy with antidepressants and none of them is free from methodological defects of various types. For all of these reasons a multi-center, double-blind clinical trial was mounted under the aegis of the Committee on Clinical Trials in Psychiatry of the Medical Research Council of Great Britain. As the details of the study have been published elsewhere (Mindham et al. 1973, see also Chapter 1), only its outline need be described here.

METHOD

The trial was conducted in eight centers in different parts of Great Britain. It was confined to patients of either sex between the ages of twenty-five and sixty-nine inclusive, all of whom were suffering from a primary depressive illness characterized by a persistent alteration in mood (with or without diurnal variation) which was evident to the examiner, which exceeded normal sadness, and which constituted a major symptom. This was supported by one or more of the following symptoms: self-depreciation with a morbid sense (or delusional ideas) of guilt; sleep disturbance; hypochondriasis; retardation of thought and action; agitated behavior. The depression was the primary illness and did not constitute merely a secondary manifestation of some other psychiatric illness (such as schizophrenia or obsessional states). Patients were excluded if they suffered from an associated progressive disease, or from any indication of structural cerebral disease, or from a physical disease which would preclude the use of amitriptyline or imipramine. Benign uncomplicated hypertension was not a contraindication. These criteria were intentionally the same as those used in a previous large-scale multicenter investigation conducted under the same auspices, which had compared the value of various forms of treatment of depression (Medical Research Council 1965).

The design of the study comprised the random allocation of eligible patients, who had responded satisfactorily to tricyclic antidepressant medication, to one of two regimens of continuation therapy. These two regimens were: (1) the same drug in a dosage of 75-150 mg daily, or (2) a placebo of identical appearance, for a period of six months. The patient and the psychiatrist were both kept unaware of which regimen had been allocated. The initial treatment consisted of either amitriptyline or imipramine in a dosage of at least 150 mg daily for between three and ten weeks. Provided that this treatment had been administered, the patients could have been treated as inpatients, outpatients, or both. In addition, it was stipulated that the patients should have received no other psychotropic drug treatment (apart from night sedation) during the final three weeks of the initial phase of their treatment, and no electroconvulsive therapy during the previous two months. For admission to the trial the patients had to have exhibited a "maximum response" to this regime—namely, an equivocal and sustained subjective and objective improvement with no evidence of further amelioration.

Patients were assessed at the start of continuation therapy and on six subsequent occasions at intervals of about one month. If, during this period, the patient suffered a further depressive episode which, in the opinion of the psychiatrist, required specific treatment, then continuation therapy was stopped and the psychiatrist started the treatment of his choice. The criterion for the effectiveness of continuation therapy was the relative frequency of such relapses in the two series.

RESULTS

A total of ninety-two patients were admitted to the trial, fifty being allocated to continuation therapy with active drugs and forty-two to the placebo. Of the many detailed findings which were recorded and analyzed about the patients and their responses to treatment, only three will be presented.

First, as Figure 13-1 demonstrates, the broad characteristics of the two treatment groups were closely similar.

Second, by the end of the period of continuation therapy, 22 percent of the patients on active treatment

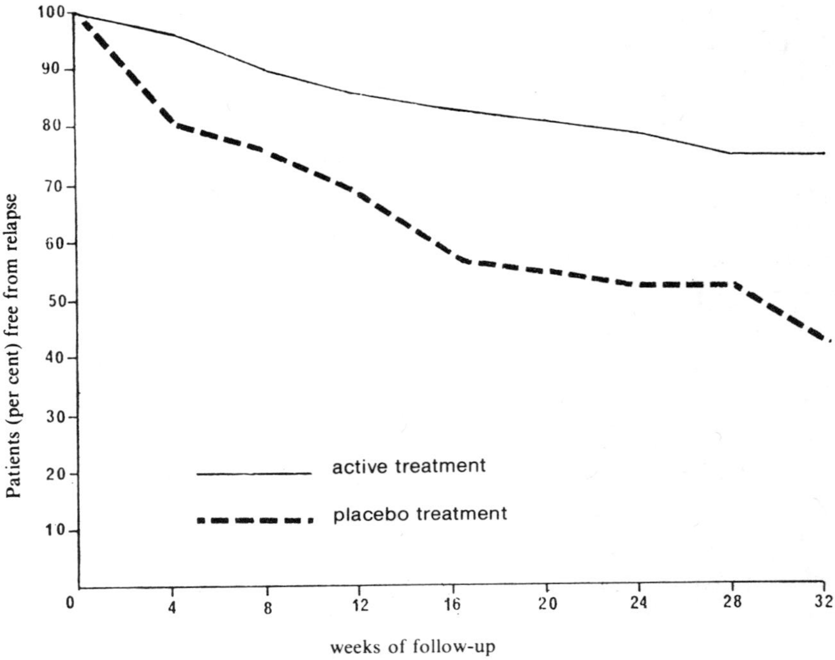

Figure 13-1. Percentages of patients remaining free from relapse in the two trial groups at four-week intervals (calculated by standard actuarial methods).

had relapsed, compared with 50 percent of those receiving placebo, a statistically significant difference. The percentages of patients remaining free of relapse in the two series at four-weekly intervals is shown in Table 13-1.

A detailed analysis of the factors which may have been associated with the differential relapse rate (Table 13-2) showed that those patients who reported residual symptoms following response to initial treatment did much better on continuation therapy with the antidepressants compared with those who received the placebo; this difference was not apparent between groups of patients with residual symptoms receiving the active and inert preparations.

DISCUSSION

Two major questions concerning the study may be singled out for comment. First, it is important to view the findings of the study in the broader perspective of antidepressant medication of depressive disorders as a whole. How representative, in short, are the results? Here it must be pointed out that the patients accepted for the trial had already responded well to an antidepressant.

Table 13-1
Comparison of the Two Treatment Series at the Start of Continuation Therapy

Characteristic	Active: No. of Subjects	Active: % of total (50)	Active: Mean Value	Placebo: No. of Subjects	Placebo: % of total (42)	Placebo: Mean Value
General:						
Male	17	**34**	—	16	**38**	—
Female	33	**66**	—	26	**62**	—
Mean age (years)	—	—	45.8	—	—	**48.3**
Earlier depressive episodes:						
None	30	**60**	—	24	**57**	—
As outpatient only	8	**16**	—	8	**19**	—
With hospital admission	12	**24**	—	10	**24**	—
Present depressive episode:						
Initial severity: Severely ill (rating 4 or 5)	11	**22**	—	11	**26**	—
(Psychiatrist) Mean rating (on scale 0—5)	—	—	3.2	—	—	**3.2**
Treatment: Electroconvulsive therapy	0	**0**	—	0	**0**	—
Amitriptyline	34	**68**	—	27	**64**	—
Imipramine	16	**32**	—	15	**36**	—
Mean duration (weeks)	—	—	7.5	—	—	7.5
Mean maximum daily dosage (mg)	—	—	166.0	—	—	175.0
Where treated: As outpatient	28	**56**	—	17	**40**	—
Mean weeks in hospital (inpatients only)	—	—	5.0	—	—	**4.4**
Severity at response date (Psychiatrist): Well (rating 0)	32	**64**	—	18	**43**	—
Minimal (rating 1)	14	**28**	—	19	**45**	—
Mean rating (on scale 0—5)	—	—	**0.5**	—	—	0.7

Table 13-2
Relapse rates in various subgroups of patients

		Active			Placebo		
		No. of Subjects	Relapsed No.	%	No. of Subjects	Relapsed No.	%
All patients		50	11	**22**	42	21	**50**
Treatment centres:	London	21	4	**19**	15	8	**53**
	Glasgow	16	3	**19**	15	4	**27**
	Elsewhere	13	4	**31**	12	9	**75**
Sex	Male	17	2	**12**	16	8	**50**
	Female	33	9	**27**	26	13	**50**
Earlier depressive episodes:	None	30	8	**27**	24	11	**46**
	As outpatient only	8	0	**0**	8	4	**50**
	With hospital admission	12	3	**25**	10	6	**60**
Present depressive episode:							
Initial severity	Severely ill (rating 4 or 5)	11	3	**27**	11	7	**64**
(Psychiatrist)	Not severely ill	39	8	**21**	31	14	**45**
Where treated:	As outpatient	28	6	**21**	17	10	**59**
	With hospital admission	22	5	**23**	25	11	**44**
Active treatment:	Amitriptyline	34	8	**24**	27	18	**67**
	Imipramine	16	3	**19**	15	3	**20**
Severity at response date: (Psychiatrist)	Well (rating 0)	32	6	**19**	18	6	**33**
	Not completely well	18	5	**28**	24	15	**62**
Symptoms at response date:	No symptoms	30	7	**23**	16	4	**25**
(Patient)	Symptoms	20	4	**20**	26	17	**65**

However, although the investigation was not concerned with the initial response to treatment, it is relevant to mention that 56 percent of the 211 patients deemed eligible for initial treatment failed to show a satisfactory response to treatment and were therefore excluded from the study. In this connection it is also relevant to recall some pertinent findings from the original Medical Research Council trial of four treatments of depressive illnesses (Medical Research Council 1965). There the illnesses were defined in identical clinical terms, although they were probably somewhat more severe, since the whole population was composed of inpatients. While the design of the earlier trial was inevitably different, only about one-third of the patients treated with tricyclic antidepressant medication at that time made a satisfactory response after twelve weeks and remained well for the subsequent three months of the study. However, as the comparable figure for patients receiving placebo was approximately one-fifth, the proportion of true drug-responders can be estimated as no more than about 15 percent of the total group treated.

Second, how effective is antidepressant medication even within these limits? Although the results of this study indicate that in terms of clinical benefit some advantage attaches to continuation therapy with tricyclic antidepressant drugs after recovery from a depressive illness, it should also be emphasized that many patients relapsed while receiving the active preparation, and that a substantial proportion of patients on the placebo remained well. As far as they go, the data support the hypothesis that the action of the antidepressant drugs that were tested is to suppress depressive symptoms rather than to relieve a postulated underlying disorder. However, a full explanation of the recorded relapse-rates would also have to take account of two other possibilities: (1) it might be that the blanket term *depressive illness* includes a number of heterogeneous conditions; and (2) some of these might be more related to nonspecific factors such as the milieu in which treatment was prescribed, the patient's social circumstances or the attitudes of individual physicians. The variation in results from the centers furnishing information serves to favor the role of this factor, but neither of these hypotheses can be treated directly by a study of this type.

It is quite clear that a great deal more work along these lines will be required before we are able to be certain of the place of continuation therapy with tricyclic drugs in the management of depressive disorders. Until that time we must remain cautious about our ability to prevent the affective illnesses.

REFERENCES

Blackwell, B. and Shepherd, M. (1968). Prophylactic lithium: another therapeutic myth? Lancet 1:968.

Freedman, A.M., Kaplan, H.I., and Sadock, B.J. (1972). Glossary of psychiatric terminology. In *Modern Synopsis of Comprehensive Textbook of Psychiatry,* p. 778. Baltimore: Williams and Wilkins.

Medical Research Council (1965). Report by clinical psychiatry committee: clinical trial of the treatment of depressive illness. *British Medical Journal* 1:881.

Mindham, R.H.S., Howland, C., and Shepherd, M. (1973). An evaluation of continuation therapy with tricyclic antidepressants in depressive illness. *Psychological Medicine* 3:5.

Wechsler, H., Grosser, G.H., and Greenblatt, M. (1965). Research evaluating antidepressant medications on hospitalized mental patients: a survey of published reports during a five-year period. *Journal of Nervous and Mental Disease* 141:231.

Part III

Social Implications

Chapter 14

The Use and Abuses of Drugs in Psychiatry

The several factors that bear on the use and abuse of drugs in psychiatry may be grouped for convenience into four overlapping categories: (1) the drugs that are used and abused; (2) the users; and (3) the abusers of them (i.e. both doctors and patients); and (4) the social milieu in which their use and abuse take place.

THE DRUGS

A large literature has already accumulated about psychotropic substances (Shepherd et al. 1968) and only two points need be underlined about the drugs themselves. The first is that the spectrum of drugs already available to the psychiatrist is a very broad one which extends, functionally, well beyond the pharmacotherapy of mental disorder. Some of the uses to which psychotropic drugs may be put were discussed in some detail at a recent conference entitled, significantly, "Manipulating and Controlling Human Behavior by Drugs—Present and Future." At this conference, one of the speakers included in his list—in addition to the formal treatment of mental illness—mental stimulation and the counteraction of fatigue; the relief of pain and the induction of pleasure; the modification of appetite, sleep, sexuality and cognitive functioning; the deliberate induction of abnormal or unusual mental states, and the alteration of psychomotor performance and aggressive conduct.

It is also becoming apparent that the capacity of many psychotropic drugs to induce adverse reactions, including dependence, is much greater than had been appreciated. A recent report of the United Nations Commission on Narcotic Drugs, for example, devoted particular attention to the importance of what is called "psychotropic substances not under international control," which included a large number of such widely prescribed drugs as the amphetamines, barbiturates, hallucinogens and tranquilizers (Commission on Narcotic Drugs 1969). In addition, there is an increasing concern about the potential risk of addiction to nonbarbiturate sedatives and several of the so-called "minor tranquilizing drugs" (Essig 1969). The World Health Organization, through its Expert Committee on Drug Dependence, is currently involved with this issue.

THE DOCTORS

In his role of physician the psychiatrist tends to regard drugs in primarily therapeutic terms. At the same time it is necessary to recognize and acknowledge a situation peculiar to this branch of medicine: namely the view that the use of drugs in itself constitutes an abuse of treatment. The origins of this viewpoint are clearly evident in the pronouncements of Pinel, whose advocacy of moral treatment was accompanied by an attitude toward physical treatment which may be illustrated by his comment that "the writings of Plato, Seneca and other writers of antiquity were found to be of more eminent service in the prevention of insanity than any pharmaceutical formulae." It may be doubted whether many modern psychiatrists are now sufficiently familiar with the classics to employ them for therapeutic purposes, but there is nevertheless a contemporary body of opinion sympathetic to Pinel's attitude toward pharmacotherapy. A number of studies, for example, have shown that practicing doctors are inclined to use and value psychotropic drugs in relation to their expressed attitudes, particularly toward psychological treatment (Haefner et al. 1960; Rose and Esser 1960). One of our more thoughtful psychotherapists has spoken of the "psychotropic effect of the doctor-patient relationship" (Kraüpl-Taylor unpublished), and recently a book entitled, *The Treatment of Mental Illness* 1969 was published with a subtitle of *Science, Faith and the Therapeutic Personality.* Among their conclusions, the authors of this book suggest that "It seems likely that patients treated with drugs in hospital will, because of their doctor's faith in them as effective remedies, learn to use them in emotional crises, and will continue to do so on discharge. In other words, they will come to look upon their own emotional reactions as symptoms of a physically determined illness, and will treat them accordingly" (Caine and Smail).

On the whole this point of view is still confined to a small but vociferous minority of psychiatrists. The great majority have not hestitated to utilize the numerous psychotropic drugs that have recently flooded the market in such quantity as to lead one student of therapeutic fashions to speak of "the great age of commercialized psychiatric treatment" (Tourney 1967). Whether many of these substances justify the claims advanced on their behalf remains, in my own view, an open question (Shepherd 1969). Meanwhile, their more enthusiastic advocates must be aware of the adverse effects of many of the psychotropic drugs if they are to avoid the charge of misuse, which the American Medical Asssociation Committee on Alcoholism and Addiction defined as "the physician's role in establishing a potentially dangerous type of therapy—even though it does not always lead to tolerance or physical dependence" (American Medical Association Committee on Alcoholism and Addiction and Council on Mental Health 1965). The Committee provided the following four examples of the misuse of sedatives: (1) prolonged and unsupervised administration of these drugs for symptomatic relief; (2) accession to a patient's demands for increased quantities of drugs, often due to a developing state of tolerance; (3) transfer from barbiturates to newer compounds in the mistaken belief of safety from abuse; and (4) the writing of repeated prescriptions without regard to possible accululative effects, additive action with other drugs, or the establishment of psychological or physical dependence.

These problems clearly confront all practicing physicians in some measure. Separate mention, however, must be made of the role of the physician whose interest in these drugs is primarily investigative rather than therapeutic. The moral problems raised by the experimental administration of compounds with so many implications for human behavior are now acknowledged in many institutions by the setting up of special committees concerned with the ethical aspects of such administration. A detailed discussion of the many legal, administrative and philosophical—as well as medical—issues involved may be found in the proceedings of a recent symposium on *Ethical Aspects of Experimentation with Human Subjects,* held under the auspices of the American Academy of Arts and Sciences. In this symposium one important, but delicate, aspect of the experimental physician's interest in therapeutic innovation was not ignored. "There can be little question," said one distinguished contributor, "that personal ambition, usually for career advancement or public acclaim, underlies much intense motivation in research work and in the trial of new ideas, drugs, operations or treatment. Such personal ambition is usually well hidden under the sophisticated affect of the dedicated clinical scientist . . . and," he continued rather unexpectedly, "far from being remiss, is the sign of a healthy society" (Moore 1969).

It could be that since the speaker was both a surgeon and an American he may have been referring to practices foreign to psychiatrists who work in less healthy societies. Nonetheless, some dedicated clinical psychopharmacologists are capable of going to considerable lengths without disturbing their sophisticated affects. By way of an example, I would mention a recent prospective study designed to investigate the relations between certain centrally acting drugs and the distressing state of dyskinesia associated with high doses of some compounds in a population of chronic schizophrenics. As might have been expected, the study demonstrated no more than a positive relationship between the incidence of dyskinesia and dosage of drug administered. More to the point, however, is that this study was submitted to a scientific journal and that one of its assessors was roused to draw a parallel between it and what passed for medical research in the concentration camps of World War II. The responsibility for setting standards in this difficult sphere of study cannot devolve on any one group of individuals but as Rutstein has emphasized, editors and editorial boards of journals that publish scientific reports of human experiments do now constitute an important instrument for scientific despumation. His conclusion is surely unexceptionable: "If higher scientific standards of publication were established and adhered to, it would soon become clear to investigators that there would be small likelihood that improperly designed studies would be published "(Rutstein 1969).

THE PATIENTS

If the doctor is liable to misuse psychotropic drugs, the patient is prone to self-abuse, a term in which psychiatrists have long displayed a professional interest. This activity is partly abetted by the medical profession. Hypnotics and sedatives are known to be the drugs most commonly prescribed by general practitioners, and Sir Derrick Dunlop has often referred to the fact that approximately 15 percent of all prescriptions written in Britain in recent years have been for psychotropic drugs. It is difficult to establish the medical criteria employed to justify this practice, but in a society where the voice of the consumer has become increasingly clamant, some attention should be paid to a point underlined recently by the Bishop of Chester, who stated that "patients regard their doctor as a kind of grocer who will deal out to them the pills which they think they need."

But even if patients do not receive satisfaction from their medical grocers they can still resort to self-medication, with all its attendant risks of abuse. The extent of, and reasons for, self-medication constitute a neglected subject of interest and importance. Some years ago, for example, we interviewed a group of patients on the list of a general practitioner. We discovered that whether or not they were attending their doctor for a medical complaint, more than 80 percent of our subjects indulged in some form of self-medication (Kessel and Shepherd 1965). In order of frequency the reasons given for taking the drugs were pain, bowel disorders, coughs and colds, indigestion, and "nerves." Sedation was mentioned infrequently, but a pharmacological breakdown showed that after aspirin, various sedatives made up the next most frequently taken class of substance. Clearly the foundations for drug dependence are being laid all around us.

SOCIETY

A former British Home Secretary has listed four "related but distinguishable issues" confronting the members of any drug-using society; these are: (1) the medical-social question, comprising the "technical aspects of the matter"; (2) the criminal law and the legal questions connected with enforcement; (3) the need for international comity; and, (4) what the Secretary was pleased to refer to as "the over-riding political judgement" (Hogg 1969).

Although this is not the place to discuss the three latter and very large topics, it may be pointed out that a fair sample of political judgement is to be found in the recent debates in the House of Commons on cannabis and in the House of Lords on drug dependence and misuse. The relevant numbers of Hansard are filled with instructive examples, including the following opinion on the careful, balanced and informed report submitted by Lady Wooton and her committee on cannabis: "I am not prepared to put to my constituents the sophisticated academic drivel in this Report. I say that with great respect, but legislation should be done by legislators, and legislators should be subject to the strict discipline of frequent election and rejection by the electorate. Although from time to time we may ask the advice of medical men and—God help us—the odd sociologist, we ought to look at it with the greatest possible skepticism" (Iremonger 1969).

In the light of such pronouncements it may be prudent for the physician to stick close to his last, but he cannot ignore the many social aspects of our knowledge about drugs, doctors and patients, to some of which I have already referred. One more point, however, needs to be emphasized at the present time. Although the market has been flooded with new psychotropic agents for the past fifteen years there is general agreement that major problems in the research and development of these substances have still to be solved. Some of these problems relate to difficulties of method and organization, but others involve wider legal, financial, and administrative issues. My own attention was drawn forcibly to these matters when our attempts to study a new antidepressant drug, supplied by an English subsidiary of a large American firm, were abruptly terminated when submission of the drug to the American Food and Drug Administration was withdrawn because of supposedly adverse effects reported elsewhere (Blackwell and Shepherd 1967). Trivial as this example may be in itself, it assumes more significance against the background of the difficulties which the powerful American pharmaceutical industry is currently experiencing with the FDA. The international ripples of this debate are well illustrated by the suggestion advanced by an American legal authority that

> The industry . . . shift[s] an increasing volume of drug research and development to foreign parts, especially to Britain, France, Germany and Italy. Costs are lower there, and controls less restrictive. Once a drug has been accepted abroad and tested in clinical experience, the process of satisfying the FDA requirements is not only easier but more certain. If American consumers were to complain of having to wait several years for drugs available abroad, no doubt the American firms could remind them that the foreigners must run the gauntlet of clinical trials. If this failed to assuage the complainants, the companies could suggest that their patrons demand that Congress lower the barriers to speedier, less expensive drug testing in this country. [Cavers 1969]

The large and growing number of new psychotropic drugs stand witness to the implications of such a proposal. The problem, however, must be tackled by conventional means, for neither the chemist's ingenuity nor the clinician's acumen has enabled us to improve on Thomas Carlyle's verdict: "Brothers, I am sorry I have got no Morrison's pill for curing the maladies of society."

REFERENCES

American Medical Association Committee on Alcoholism and Addiction and Council on Mental Health (1965). Dependence on barbiturates and other sedative drugs. *Journal of the American Medical Association* 193:673-677.

Blackwell, B., and Shepherd, M. (1967). Early evaluation of psychotropic drugs in man. *Lancet* 2:819-822.

Caine, T.M., and Smail, D.J. (1969), *The Treatment of Mental Illness,* University of London Press, p. 169.

Cavers, D.F. (1969). Ethical aspects of experimentation with human subjects. *Daedalus: Journal of the American Academy of Arts and Sciences,* p. 433. Boston: American Academy of Arts and Sciences.

Commission on Narcotic Drugs (1969). Report of the Twenty-third Session, New York, p. 62.

Essig, C.F. (1969). The potential risk of addiction to nonbarbiturate sedative and minor tranquilizing drugs. In *Abuse of Central Stimulants,* ed. F. Sjöqvist and M. Tottie, p. 89. Stockholm: Almquist and Wiksell Forlag AB.

Haefner, D.P., Sacks, J.M., and Mason, A.S. (1960). Physicians' attitudes toward chemotherapy as a factor in psychiatric patients' responses to medication. *Journal of Nervous and Mental Disease* 131:64-69.

Hogg, Q. (1969). Parliamentary debates (Hansard), 776, number 4, p. 950. London: Her Majesty's Stationery Office.

Iremonger, T.L. (1969). Parliamentary debates (Hansard), 776, number 4, p. 995. London: Her Majesty's Stationery Office.

Kessel, N., and Shepherd, M. (1965), The health and attitudes of people who seldom consult a doctor. *Medical Care* 3:6-10.

Kraupl-Taylor, F. (Unpublished). *Comments on the Postgraduate Training in Psychiatry.*

Moore, F.D. (1969). Ethical aspects of experimentation with human subjects. *Daedalus: Journal of the American Academy of Arts and Sciences,* p. 518. Boston: American Academy of Arts and Sciences.

Rose, M., and Esser, M.A. (1960). The impact of recent research developments on private practice. *American Journal of Psychiatry* 117:429-433.

Rutstein, D.D. (1969). Ethical aspects of experimentation with human subjects. *Daedalus: Journal of the American Academy of Arts and Sciences,* p. 525. Boston: American Academy of Arts and Sciences.

Shepherd, M. (1969). Therapeutic problems with psychotropic drugs: some epidemiological considerations. *Psychiatria, Neurologia and Neurochirurgia* 72:503-506.

Shepherd, M., Lader, M.H. and Rodnight, R. (1968). *Clinical Psychopharmacology.* London: English Universities Press.

Tourney, G. (1967). A history of therapeutic fashions in psychiatry, 1800-1966. *American Journal of Psychiatry.* 124:784-796.

Chapter 15

Transcultural Approaches to the Treatment of Mental Disorder

If it is true, as Gaddum (1959) has maintained, that "the most important changes in medicine during this century have been due to advances in knowledge of methods for the prevention and cure of disease," then the psychiatrist must take a modest view of progress within his specialty. Although psychiatry has been able to draw traditionally on physical, psychological and environmental methods of treatment, rational therapeutic achievement, based on an understanding of the etiology of illness, remains confined to a small segment of the whole large area of mental disorder. Empiricism, which lends itself so readily to dogma and opinion, has dominated therapeutics and even a cursory review of national practices shows there to be greater variation in psychiatry than in most other branches of medicine.

In some measure this diversity reflects lack of knowledge. More is known about the genesis of many medical and surgical diseases than about all but a few psychiatric disorders. Where the facts are best established, as with general paralysis or the myxedematous psychoses, there is broad agreement on the principles of treatment. Ignorance of physical causation, however, accounts only in part for the wide national differences in psychiatric practice.

The growing appreciation of the role of socioenvironmental factors in psychiatric illness endorses the conclusion of the chairman of the American Psychiatric Association's Committee on International Relations, that: "in psychiatry . . . the physician intercedes between, not only man and nature, but most often and mainly, between man and society" (Galdston 1957). In consequence, the comparative method, to which Kraepelin drew attention nearly sixty years ago as a means of investigating psychopathological and epidemiological phenomena in psychiatry (Kraepelin 1904), can also be expected to illuminate the problems of therapy. The method can do this by specifically identifying social treatments in different cultures and subcultures, and by delineating the implicit or explicit role of sociocultural factors in the choice of forms of treatment. Systematic investigation in this field has been handicapped by a dearth of reliable data; nonetheless, it has seemed most profitable to remain close to the few factual landmarks, and to avoid whenever possible the overgrown thicket of impressions and generalizations.

THE PSYCHIATRIC HOSPITAL

The psychiatric hospital would, at first sight, appear a convenient point of departure, since the development of formal treatment for the major psychoses has been closely associated with institutions and the people attached to them. The psychiatric hospital, however, symbolizes socioeconomic development, as well as a certain stage of medicosocial awareness of the needs of the mentally ill (Jones 1960), and international comparisons of psychiatric practice are futile without regarding the development of the medical services of individual countries. In economically depressed countries with a low standard of living, the level of psychiatric training cannot be detached from the efficacy of the public health service; where such disorders as malnutrition, trypanosomiasis and encephalitis are endemic, each has its psychiatric complications. Pacheco e Silva (1960), referring to the dimensions of this problem in Latin America, has pointed out that much psychiatric morbidity must be regarded as an integral part of the socioeconomic and political environment that leads to and maintains ill health. Furthermore, in some nations, specialized psychiatric resources for the management of even the graver mental diseases may be quite inadequate by the standards of more affluent societies. The Indian State of Mysore, for example, contains one 300-bed hospital to serve more than nine million people (Hoenig and Srinivasan 1959), whereas Denmark, with well over half this population, has eight mental hospitals with more than 7,000 beds among them (Aungle 1958). Similarly, what Albee (1960) refers to as a manpower crisis in mental health in the United States—where there are more than 10,000 trained psychiatrists—takes on a different perspective when it is recalled that huge areas in Africa can claim no more than a handful of physicians.

Under these conditions, treatment becomes primarily a matter of communal activity rather than of hospital care. Ethnopsychiatric studies in many parts of the world have shown both the importance of community attitudes towards the mentally ill (World Health Organization 1960), and of the local measures taken to support them. Four illustrations make the point. Lambo (1959) has emphasized that "hospitals are viewed with deep suspicion in Africa and consequently patients are usually seen or brought at a crucial stage of their illness when all other measures have failed"; he has, accordingly, based an effective community-care program in Aro, Western Nigeria, on the village system with a day hospital. In Sierra Leone, Maclay (unpublished) has observed that patients whose conduct is too difficult for family care are often kept in the community and given local native treatment;" they can be found with their legs confined in stocks and may be cruelly ill-treated; on the other hand, the chronic harmless types seem to be accepted and are cared for in much the same way as the 'village idiot' used to be in England." Manugian (1958) has related the Moslem and Druze religious teachings in Lebanon to the respect and protection afforded in that country to old people, who are often kept at home even when suffering from advanced senile psychoses. And, lastly, mention should be made of the use of indigenous medicaments, such as the Rauwolfia plant in India and southern Iran, whose potential value is only now being subjected to scientific investigation.

PENOLOGY AND PSYCHIATRY

Where it is to be found in economically less advanced countries, the psychiatric hospital often assumes a function which is more custodial than therapeutic, serving chiefly, as Tooth (1950) has observed of the Gold Coast, "to protect the public from dangerous and criminal lunatics." In many societies the institutional treatment of antisocial conduct by abnormal members of society is linked to the juristic concept of social defense; and as the law mirrors a nation's political and moral values, so its practitioners tend to disagree even more readily than physicians on the psychiatric treatment of offenders. The differences between national criminal codes and their relationship to therapeutic practice go beyond the scope of this review. It may suffice to cite the comment of one authority on European legislation concerning the penal status of such deviant sexual behavior as homosexuality, incest and bestiality: "although the sexual drive is one of the basic instincts of man and its manifestations one of the most usual, there is perhaps no ground on which ethical and legal views differ so widely on the border between the licit and the illicit even among peoples at the same historical period and at the same state of civilization" (Antoliesi 1955). It was therefore to be expected that, despite much discussion on the relative merits of therapeutic measures conducted in mental hospitals, penal institutions, psychiatric prisons and "in freedom," Gibbens's careful (1950) comparison of several experiments in institutional care should have led him to conclude that these could "only be judged in relation to the social and legal systems in which they operate."

In his review of the management of abnormal offenders in sixteen European countries, Cornil (1956) has outlined the wide variations in methods of detection, the factors influencing court decisions, and the principles of treatment. He has suggested that the concept of the abnormal offense is itself unclear from both the legal and the psychiatric standpoints, and that in most countries it is still bound up with the notion of criminal responsibility. Confusion of thought and division of opinion are most marked with regard to the "*demi-fous* . . . the intermediate group of offenders suffering from a less serious form of mental disorder but not completely responsible for their actions and qualifying for mitigation of their penalty."

As the definition of illness becomes less precise, the old dilemma of sickness or sin raises the complementary issue of therapy or correction, a problem which tends to be resolved by sociopolitical as well as by medicolegal principles. Most Western societies accept in principle

Glueck's (1954) view of the antisocial individual as "a sick person, in need of treatment rather than punishment"; for example, a psychopathic disorder, according to the British Mental Health Act of 1959, by definition "requires or is susceptible to medical treatment." This attitude, however, differs sharply from a recent statement of the current Russian position: "as we believe that upbringing plays the decisive role in shaping a person's character, we consequently, as a rule, recognize psychopaths as responsible individuals—that is to say as standing in need of judicial reformative influence, rather than medical care" (Popov 1958). The dialectic consequences of this premise, that: "the educative role of the social environment . . . explains why a comparatively insignificant percentage of psychopaths in the Soviet Union are delinquents," remains to be demonstrated. Meanwhile, it is clear that the modern psychopath, as the "linguistic descendant of the old 'moral defective' " (Wootton 1959), continues to pose therapeutic problems which cannot be elucidated in strictly medical terms when social groups are compared.

METHODS OF TREATMENT

Forensic considerations apart, the growth of psychiatric institutions has undoubtedly facilitated the development of most procedures which have been employed in the treatment of the major psychoses. Universal agreement on the broad principles of therapy, however, extends to very few conditions, all of them with a clearly defined physical basis. About the many empirical forms of treatment which are in use for the functional psychoses, there are numerous and often conflicting opinions. National preferences cannot be explained wholly in terms of the proven merits or shortcomings of these procedures. Certain trends can be detected, as in the conclusion of a recent American report on the treatment of the mentally ill in Europe, that: "treatment procedures are more organically orientated than they are in the United States" (Casey et al. 1960). A general verdict of this type, however, does less than justice to the diversity of national patterns. It does not explain why the Dutch have concentrated on administrative measures designed to treat patients out of hospital (Lemkau and Crocetti 1961); why the intensive psychotherapy of schizophrenia has found so much favor in some Swiss and German centers; why deep insulin-therapy has waned more rapidly in England than in Austria; why sleep-treatment has been carried out so energetically in some French hospitals; or why the elimination of focal sepsis can occasionally remain an objective in the mid-twentieth century (Harris 1949). Nor does it account for the ukase on prefrontal leucotomy in the USSR and the low status of electroconvulsive therapy in that country (Lustig 1958).

The complex nature of the forces which determine the choice or rejection of a specific form of treatment in psychiatric institutions has been illustrated in the past decade by the reception given to the newer psychotropic drugs. The therapeutic claims made on behalf of these compounds have created a widespread interest in the possibilities of pharmacotherapy. The drugs have been prescribed extensively in most countries which can afford them, and some hospitals have virtually discarded other forms of physical treatment. On the other hand, the pharmacodynamic action of these substances is poorly understood and the results of controlled investigations have already modified the more extravagant early pronouncements (Foulds 1958). There is also some statistical evidence to suggest that drug treatment has proved most effective when the preceding level of institutional care has been low (Shepherd et al. 1961). A number of studies have shown a relationship between response to chemotherapy and the attitudes of psychiatric physicians (Haefner et al. 1960), who are divided among themselves about the value of individual compounds. A recent survey of American views succeeded only in demonstrating "the diversity of opinion regarding the usefulness of the drugs and the variability of techniques in their utilization" (Margolis 1959). The attractions of a conventionally "medical" form of physical treatment in place of the cruder alternatives appears to be balanced by an interest in the possibilities of social therapy for patients in institutions. According to one authority, for example, "hospital administrative reforms would be crying in the wilderness if the so-called tranquilizing drugs had not appeared" (Mayer-Gross 1959); while another states flatly that "if we had to choose between abandoning the use of the new drugs and abandoning the industrial rehabilitation centers and other industrial facilities available to us there would be no hesitation about the choice; the drugs would go" (Lewis 1959). In addition, account must be taken of the energetic campaigns of the pharmaceutical industry, the influence of individual physicians, and the expectations of a public in broad agreement with Aldous Huxley's (1959) suggestion that "in a world where nobody gets anything for nothing, tranquilizers offer a great deal for very little." The climate of opinion favoring pharmacotherapy cannot then be understood without regard to many medicosocial factors (Shepherd 1961) whose interplay also contributes to other current empirical fashions.

MINOR PSYCHIATRIC DISORDERS

When we turn from the major psychoses to the minor psychiatric disabilities, it is to find that an appreciation of their distribution and nature is relatively recent, most of it coming from epidemiological research since the Second

World War. The old assertion that minor psychiatric illness occurs infrequently in less industrialized societies has been rebutted by the findings of such workers as Lin (1953) in Formosa, Eaton and Weil (1955) among the Hutterites, and Lambo (1960) in Nigeria. Lacking formal psychiatric facilities, many of these societies have evolved therapeutic methods based on faith rather than on understanding, but these can nonetheless be effective. For example, Field (1958) has examined the role of the shrines of native deities in Ghana, and Gillin (1957) has paid special attention to the process of care in cases of "magical fright" in a Guatemalan community. Gillin's description of the stages of the "curing session," which takes place only on Friday nights, is as follows:

> (1) The curer first conducts a diagnostic interview, including feeling the pulses. The patient is induced to tell his recent preoccupations, activities and dreams. If the curer decides that the patient is suffering from magical fright rather than some other condition such as bewitchment, evil eye or corpse sickness, the cure continues. The interview usually elicits a mildly cathartic "confession" from the patient. (2) Assurance is given the patient and a certain "transference" established, that is, the patient is induced to have confidence in the curer. (3) The practitioner next endeavors to assuage the physical complaints, using pharmaceutical as well as folkloristic preparations. (4) The patient is drawn from his social isolation. (5) A Principal, one of the six highest religious and civic authorities in the native community, is engaged to participate in the cure. (6) With the help of the Principal an elaborate ritual is carried out, explaining the situation to the images of the Christian saints. This is necessary to gear the cure into the Christian scheme of things because commerce must later be had with familiar spirits of the cure and renegade saints who have captured the soul. (7) An expedition is made in the middle of the night to the site of the alleged fright, where the occult captors of the soul are appealed to on a man-to-man basis by

> the curer and are provided an offering of worldly goods for their enjoyment. (8) The patient is massaged with eggs in the shell which are supposed to draw the illness out of him. The eggs are then broken in water and an augury is read in the shapes of the floating whites. Some curers use eggs as part of the diagnosis; most practitioners employ them as a magical verification of the cure. (9) The curer takes the patient naked into the chill night air at 2 A.M. and, without warning, blows from his mouth numerous blasts of magic mixture over him. This is said to blow the evil winds out of his body, but also serves as a sort of "shock treatment." (10) The patient is given a cathartic drink. (11) He is thoroughly rubbed down, wrapped in blankets and put to bed to sweat. (12) Before the patient goes to sleep a bowl of copal gum with hot coals is placed under his bed and is so manipulated by the curer that the copal bursts into flames and envelops the patient in a cloud of sweet smelling smoke (copal was the sacred incense of the ancient Maya). The flame is regarded as a sign that the soul has returned to the body. The patient usually sinks into a deep, relaxed sleep. Although he may have to get up during the night to empty his bowels, due to the cathartic administered during the curing session, he typically awakens the next day in a cheerful frame of mind and restored to his "normal" personality.

This ritual includes several elements familiar to more medically sophisticated societies, where it is equally true that "whatever the therapeutic value of the other aspects of the treatment, the sociocultural features are of great importance." In wealthier countries it is apparent that the formal process of detection, diagnosis, and treatment of neurosis cannot be divorced from the structure of the medical services, since relatively few patients suffering from minor psychiatric illness require institutional care. For one thing, the administrative and financial structure of outpatient psychiatric services varies widely from country to country. As a rule these services tend to be less systematically developed than the inpatient facilities, even in such well-organized areas as the Scandinavian bloc. In Italy, for example, the small number of Servizi di Igiene e Profilassi Mentale are confined mostly to the northern part of the country, and neurologists treat many psychiatric cases privately (Fazio 1961). In the Soviet Union, where there is virtually no private practice, most neurotic illnesses are treated by "neuropathologists" working in dispensaries (Kline 1960). By contrast, nearly two-thirds of American psychiatrists treat patients privately, with about one-fifth of them undertaking no other professional activity (Joint Information Service Fact Sheet 1959). It is equally relevant that, even in countries with elaborate social services, the general practitioner may, as in West Germany (Fish 1961), have a financial interest in retaining the patient rather than in referring him to a hospital.

As for the management of patients suffering from the neuroses and personality disorders, eclectic psychiatrists everywhere appear to agree on the value of centrally-acting drugs, psychological support or explanation, and environmental manipulation in symptomatic treatment. However, few authorities stress the role of biological therapy at the present time, and there is sharp disagreement on the emphasis to be placed on psychological and social factors in the management of these conditions. In many Western societies psychological techniques have been regarded as the treatment of choice for neuroses. Several psychotherapeutic systems have been developed, usually through the efforts of gifted individuals, but few have made more than local headway. Of the Daseinsanalyse, for example, it has been said with tart justice that " 'Being-in-the-World' . . . becomes synonymous with 'Being-in-the-Academic-World-of-Europe' " (Mayer-Gross et al. 1960). In the United States, however, Freudian psychoanalytic theory and practice has found so much favor as to engender the claim that "psychiatrists in America treat conflicts, whereas in Europe they treat symptoms" (Mora 1959).

Although psychoanalysis represents a view of psychological determinism essentially independent of social forces—despite the modification of later theorists influenced by sociological and anthropological thinking—its widespread adoption in the United States has enabled several workers to evaluate this system in its social setting. Thus Stengel (1960) has indicated its appeal to a society which prizes pragmatism above a philosophical preoccupation with psychiatric therapy; other psychiatrists have speculated on the contact of psychoanalysis with various strands in American cultural life, including the pioneering tradition, the puritan ethos, the myth of equality, and the intense, competitive need for material success (Knoepfel and Redlich 1952, 1953, Lidz and Lidz 1950). Among the most searching observations about the social context of psychiatry are those of Hollingshead and Redlich (1958), who have investigated the relationship of psychiatric treatment to the American social class structure, and who have illustrated some of their conclusions graphically with the case histories of two "compulsively promiscuous adolescent females."

> Both girls came to the attention of the police at the same time but under very different circumstances. One came from a core group class I family, the other from a class V broken by the desertion of the father. The class I girl, after one of her frequent drinking and sexual escapades on a weekend away from an exclusive boarding-school, became involved in an automobile accident while drunk. Her family immediately arranged bail through the influence of a member of an outstanding law firm; a powerful friend telephoned a newspaper contact, and the report of the accident was not published. Within twenty-four hours, the girl was returned to school. In a few weeks the school authorities

> realized the girl was pregnant and notified her parents. A psychiatrist was called in for consultation by the parents with the expectation, expressed frankly, that he was to recommend a therapeutic interruption of the pregnancy. He did not see fit to do this and, instead recommended hospitalization in a psychiatric institution to initiate psychotherapy. The parents, though disappointed that the girl would not have a "therapeutic" abortion, finally consented to hospitalization. In due course, the girl was delivered of a healthy baby who was placed for adoption. Throughout her stay in hospital she received intensive psychotherapy and after being discharged continued in treatment with a highly regarded psychoanalyst.
>
> The class V girl was arrested by the police after she was observed having intercourse with four or five sailors from a nearby naval base. At the end of a brief and perfunctory trial, the girl was sentenced to a reform school. After two years she was paroled as an unpaid domestic. While on parole, she became involved in promiscuous activity, was caught by the police and sent to the state reformatory for women. She accepted her sentence as deserved "punishment" but created enough disturbance in the reformatory to attract the attention of a guidance officer. This official recommended that a psychiatrist be consulted. The psychiatrist who saw her was impressed by her crudeness and inability to communicate with him on most subjects. He was alienated by the fact that she thought masturbation was "bad" whereas intercourse with many men whom she hardly knew was "O.K." The psychiatrist's recommendation was to return the girl to her regular routine because she was not "able to profit from psychotherapy."

The reasons for national opposition to depth psychology also have their social and cultural roots (Arieti 1952). Students of Japanese society have indicated the clash between psychoanalytic concepts and the traditional values of the East (Caudill 1959, Doi 1955). In Italy, where psychiatry has developed with a marked biological emphasis (Lemkau and de Sanctis 1950), Bazzi (1956) has argued against an explanation for this in terms of the political, religious, or economic structure of that country, coming down instead in favor of certain national characterisitcs as its crucial determinants: "Im Menschenbild Freuds oder Jungs erkennt sich der Italiener nicht." (The Italian does not recognize himself in the picture of man provided by Freud or Jung.) From Eastern Europe, the lead from the Soviet Union is explicit. In his exposition *The Ideological Struggle with Neo-freudianism* Bassin (1959) has explained that "the usefulness of compromising Pavlovian physiology with Freudianism and psychoanalysis is usually justified by the argument that only the latter explains the basis of psychological conflict and unconscious behavior. This argument is incorrect for two reasons: (1) the psychoanalytic explanation of the problem of conflict and "unconsciousness" is not based on scientific fact, in addition to being useless in therapy; and (2) the actual explanation of this problem is offered by the Pavlov school and by a series of researches carried out from the position of dialectical and materialistic psychoneurology and psychology." The nexus between this viewpoint and political theory has been pointed out by Stuchlik (1959) in relation to events in Czechoslovakia since 1948. However, those attempts made by individual workers in the Western world to apply Pavlovian theory in the treatment of neurotic illness have so far met with indifferent success (Lancet 1961), and in practice most attention to declared neurosis in Russia appears to be devoted to work-therapy, rest in sanatoria, and a form of psychotherapy," emphasizing social and environmental factors" (Kalinowski 1960), which concentrates on the need to achieve a close integration with society.

For Great Britain, as a country in which social psychiatry has been intensively developed—and which has outstanding achievements in the field of mental hospital reform to its credit—perhaps the most challenging development to outpatient psychiatry is the Soviet claim of having reduced the prevalence of psychoneurosis by prophylactic social measures so that the "low morbidity rate is officially attributed to the 'sheltered' life of the population and the complete absence of unemployment in the country" (World Health Organization 1959). The validity of this contention must be assessed against the background of a health service which differs in its essential philosophy from those of many European societies (Lancet 1959). Nonetheless, the emphasis on a communal approach to minor mental disorders is in line with the broad development epitomized in Great Britain by the Mental Health Act. The Act "assumes as its starting point that psychiatry is like any other part of medicine and that mental health services are an integral part of the health services generally" (British Medical Journal 1960). The far-reaching implications of this premise have been underlined by Fraser (1960), who has observed that emotional disturbances are "frequently the results of conditions in the home or at work and are often due to the personal relations with other members of the family, neighbors, or colleagues at the place of employment. Thus it is often difficult to distinguish between the fields of social and preventive medicine and of psychiatry." On this basis, the medical agent most closely concerned with minor psychiatric illness in a modern Welfare State is the family doctor rather than the psychiatric specialist, and it can be argued that he may be the most appropriate person to undertake treatment (Kessel and Shepherd 1962). Reshaping the practitioner's function in society, however, involves an acceptance of psychosocial problems as legitimate issues of medical concern on the part of the patient, as well as of the doctor. The process will necessitate a change in attitude by many physicians and in France, at least, there is some evidence to suggest that the public does not regard the doctor as a desirable confidant (Sondages 1960). With this proviso it should be possible for the National Health Service to foster in the community a program of psychiatric treatment which will constitute an integral part of the discipline of social medicine.

REFERENCES

Albee, G.W. (1960). The manpower crisis in mental health. *American Journal of Public Health* 50:1895.

Antoliesi, F. (1955). *Manuele di Diritto Penale.* Vol. 2. Milan.

Arieti, S. (1952). Anti-psychoanalytic cultural forces in the development of Western civilization. *American Journal of Psychotherapy* 6:63–78.

Aungle, P.G. (1958). Mental hospital planning in Denmark. *Journal of Mental Science* 104:477-82.

Bassin, F.V. (1959). The ideological struggle with neo-freudianism. *Extracta Int. Congressus Psychiatricus Bohemslovenicus,* Lazne Jesenk.

Bazzi, T. (1956). Psychotherapie in Italien. Völkerpsychologische Betrachtungen im Rahmen der psychotherapeutisches Praxis. *Zeitschrift für Psychotherapie und Medizinische Psychologie* 3:241-51.

British Medical Journal (1960). The Mental Health Act. Editorial. 2:1297.

Casey, J.F., Rackow, L.L. and Sperry, A.W. (1960). *Observations on the Treatment of the Mentally Ill in Europe.* Washington, D.C.: Veterans Administration, p. 13.

Caudill, W. (1959). Observations on the cultural context of Japanese psychiatry. In *Culture and Mental Health,* ed. M.K. Opler, pp. 213–42. London: Macmillan.

Cornil, P. (1956). *General Report on the Treatment of Abnormal Offenders.* Working Paper No. 2, European Consultative Group on the Prevention of Crime and the Treatment of Offenders. Geneva: United Nations (unpublished).

Doi, L.T. (1955). Some aspects of Japanese psychiatry. *American Journal of Psychiatry* 3:691-95.

Eaton, J.W., and Weil, R.J. (1955). *Culture and Mental Disorders.* Glencoe, Ill.: Free Press.

Fazio, C. (1961). Personal communication.

Field, M.J. (1958). Mental disorder in rural Ghana. *Journal of Mental Science* 104:1043-51.

Fish, F.J. (1961). Personal communication.

Foulds, G.A. (1958). Clinical research in psychiatry. *Journal of Mental Science* 104:259-65.

Fraser, F.R. (1960). The challenge to the medical profession. *British Medical Journal* 2:1821-26.

Gaddum, J.H. (1959). Methods and problems associated with the evaluation of drugs in man: 1. Introduction. In *Quantitative Methods in Human Pharmacology and Therapeutics*, ed. D.R. Laurence, pp. 3–10. Oxford: Pergamon Press.

Galdston, I. (1957). International psychiatry. *American Journal of Psychiatry* 114:103-08.

Gibbens, T.C.N. (1950). Recent trends in the management of psychopathic offenders. *British Journal of Delinquency* 2:1035-36.

Gillin, J. (1957). Cross-cultural aspects of socio-cultural therapy: Guatemala. In *Progress in Psychotherapy*, vol. 2, ed. J.H. Masserman and J.L. Moreno, pp. 224-30. New York: Grune and Stratton.

Glueck, B.C., Jr. (1954). Changing concepts in forensic psychiatry. *Journal of Criminal Law, Criminology and Police Science* 127:36.

Haefner, D.P., Sacks, J.M., and Mason, A.S. (1960). Physicians' attitudes towards chemotherapy as a factor in psychiatric patients' responses to medication. *Journal of Nervous and Mental Disease* 131:64-69.

Harris, A. (1949). Impressions of Scandinavian psychiatry. *Journal of Mental Science* 95:867-73.

Hoenig, J., and Srinivasan, U. (1959). Aspects of the Mental Health Service—present and past. *Journal of the All-India Institute of Mental Health* 2:13-25.

Hollingshead, A.B., and Redlich, F.C. (1958). *Social Class and Mental Illness.* New York: Wiley, p. 175.

Huxley, A. (1959). *Brave New World Revisited.* London: Chatto and Windus, p. 103.

Joint Information Service of the American Psychiatric Association and the National Association for Mental Health, (1959). Fact Sheet Number 10. Number, distribution and activities of psychiatrists. Washington, D.C.: A.P.A.

Jones, K. (1960). *Mental Health and Social Policy: 1845-1959*. London: Routledge and Kegan Paul.

Kalinowsky, L. (1960). Impressions of Soviet psychiatry. *Comprehensive Psychiatry* 1:35-41.

Kessel, W.I.N. and Shepherd, M. (1962). Neurosis in hospital and general practice. *Journal of Mental Science* 108:159.

Kline, N.S. (1960). The organization of psychiatric care and psychiatric research in the Union of Soviet Socialist Republics. *Annals of the New York Academy of Science* 84:149-223.

Knoepfel, H.K., and Redlich, F.C. (1952/53). Psychiatrische Ausbildung in U.S.A. *Psyche* 1:67-69.

Kraepelin, E. (1904). Vergleichende Psychiatrie. *Zeutralblatt der Nervenheilkunde und Psychiatrie* 27:433-37.

Lambo, T.A. (1959). A form of social psychiatry in Africa. Paper to the Permanent Inter-African Bureau for Tsetse and Trypanosomiasis, Ibadan (unpublished).

Lambo, T.A. (1960). Further neuropsychiatric observations in Nigeria. *British Medical Journal* 2:1696-704.

Lancet (1959). Looking to to-morrow. Editorial. 1:29-31.

Lancet)1961). Pavlov or Freud. Editorial. 1:492-93.

Lemkau, P.V., and de Sanctus, C. (1950). A survey of Italian psychiatry 1949. *American Journal of Psychiatry* 107:401-08.

Lemkau, P.V. and Crocetti, G.M. (1961). The Amsterdam Municipal Psychiatric Service: a psychiatric-sociological review. *American Journal of Psychiatry* 117:779-83.

Lewis, A. (1959). The impact of psychotropic drugs on the structure, function and future of psychiatric services. In *Neuropsychopharmacology*, vol. 1, ed. P.B. Bradley, P. Deniker, and C. Radouco-Thomas, pp. 207-12. Amsterdam: Elsevier.

Lidz, R.W. and Lidz, T. (1950). Eine Interpretation der Grundideen der Amerikanischen Psychiatrie. *Nervanarzt* 21:490-94.

Lin, T. (1953). A study of the incidence of mental disorders in Chinese and other cultures. *Psychiatry* 16:313-36.

Lustig, B. (1958). Uber therapeutische Methoden in der neueren sowjetischen Psychiatrie. *Fortschritte der Neurologie, Psychiatrie und Ihrer Genzgebiate* 26:209-19.

Maclay, W.S. (unpublished). *Report on Mental Health Service of Sierra Leone.*

Manugian, A.S. (1958). *General Attitudes of the Community in Respect of Abnormal Persons of Advanced Age.* Working Paper Number 19 to the World Health Organization Expert Committee on Mental Health, Geneva. (unpublished).

Margolis, L.H. (1959). Attitudes to psychotropic drugs. In *A Pharmacological Approach to the Study of the Mind,* ed. R.M. Featherstone and A. Simon. Springfield, Ill.: Thomas.

Mayer-Gross, W. (1959). Model psychoses: their history, relevancy and limitations. *American Journal of Psychiatry* 115:673-82.

Mayer-Gross, W., Slater, E.T.O., and Roth, M. (1960). *Clinical Psychiatry.* London: Cassell, p. 30.

Mora, G. (1959). Recent American psychiatric developments (since 1939). In *American Handbook of Psychiatry,* vol. 1. ed. S. Arieti. New York: Basic Books.

Pacheco e Silva, A.A. (1960). Mental hygiene in underdeveloped countries. *Revista Archives de Neurologia y Psychiatria* 10:5-15.

Popov, E.A. (1958). *The Forensic Problems Presented by Psychopaths.* Paper for World Health Organization Seminar on the Psychiatric Treatment of Criminals and Delinquents, Copenhagen (unpublished).

Shepherd, M. (1961). The present status of psychopharmacology.*Journal of Chronic Diseases* 13:289-92.

Shepherd, M., Goodman, N. and Watt, D.C. (1961). The application of hospital statistics in the evaluation of pharmacotherapy in a psychiatric population. *Comprehensive Psychiatry* 2:11-19.

Sondages, Revue Francaise de L'Opinion Publique (1960). *Les Francais et Leur Medicine* Numbers 1 and 2.

Stengel, E. (1960). Neurosenprobleme von anglo-amerikanischen Geischtspunkt. In *Psychiatrie der Gegenwart,* vol. 2, ed. H.W. Gruhle, R. Jung, W. Mayer-Gross, and M. Müller, pp. 203-13. Berlin: Springer Verlag.

Stuchlik, J. (1959). On the development and present state of psychotherapy in Czechoslovakia. In *Progress in Psychotherapy,* vol. 9, ed. J.H Masserman, and J.L. Moreno. New York: Grune and Stratton.

Tooth, G. (1950). Studies in mental illness in the Gold Coast. *Colonial Research Publications*, Number 6:24. London: Her Majesty's Stationery Office.

World Health Organization (1959). Social psychiatry and community attitudes. *World Health Organization Technical Reprint Service* 177:Geneva.

World Health Organization (1960). Health Services in the U.S.S.R. *World Health Organization Public Health Paper* Number 3, Geneva.

Wootton, B. (1959). *Social Science and Social Pathology* London: Allen and Unwin, p. 249.

Chapter 16

Epidemiological Aspects of Psychiatric Drug Therapy

New drugs may be introduced into medical practice in one of two ways. Very rarely their adoption follows a careful process of animal testing and controlled evaluation on human subjects. Much more frequently it follows on an amalgam of clinical enthusiasm, uncontrolled impressions, and pharmaceutical promotion. And yet, paradoxically, if this latter and most unscientific process should lead to a compound or class of compounds being widely adopted, it may become possible to examine the drug's efficacy, doing this in a scientific manner by a retrospective examination of the impact of the drug on the sizable populations to which it has already been administered.

This application of the epidemiological method of inquiry has so far been applied most often to psychiatric inpatient populations, about which statistical information is readily obtainable in many countries. It was not long after the appearance of the new psychotropic drugs in the early 1950s that individual workers began to employ this method in support of their claims for therapeutic action of such drugs. Probably the most influential of these reports came from New York State, where Brill and Patton (1959) pointed out that the arrival of large scale pharmacotherapy had coincided with a sharp fall in the number of hospitalized persons and a corresponding rise in the number of discharges. Similar trends were recorded by the national mental hospital statistics of the United Kingdom and led to similar assumptions about causation. On the other hand, it was also quickly realized that any adequate explanation of the crude statistics had also to take into account a host of nonspecific factors which contribute to the ambience of hopeful enthusiasm that accompanies any novel therapeutic procedure. If such factors were to play a significant role, it would follow that the impact of psychotropic drugs, as reflected by the population dynamics, would be much smaller in institutions in which a high degree of patient care had already been attained. To examine this hypothesis we were able, some years ago, to carry out an intensive study of one of the better English mental hospitals. We did this over a period of four years extending from 1954, the year preceding the introduction of the drugs, to 1957, by which time the drugs were being widely prescribed (Shepherd et al. 1961). We were able to demonstrate that a marked improvement, in terms of a higher discharge rate and a shorter hospital stay, had already taken place ten years earlier, long before the appearance of psychotropic drugs, and that this change was probably due to a combination of the somatic treatments of that time allied to an unusually progressive mental health service.

A study of the type we carried out depends on a complex statistical analysis of a number of factors. These include the average annual numbers of patients in different diagnostic categories who were resident, admitted, or discharged; the mortality rate, "quittance-rate," and "net release rate"; and the numbers of patients receiving various quantities of psychotropic drugs during the survey period. The detailed results of our study were presented in the original publication. Here it need only be said that our findings, in terms of the resident population and the psychiatric admissions from 1954 to 1958, showed that, in the event, every little change was recorded.

Our suggested explanation, based on a knowledge of the local situation, was that before the new psychotropic drugs were introduced this hospital was functioning as part of an effective mental health service which had already taken up the therapeutic slack. Clearly, such an hypothesis becomes immeasurably strengthened if it can be reinforced by comparable findings elsewhere. It was therefore gratifying to observe the very similar findings published later by Ödegaard, who had independently analyzed the mental hospital statistics of Norway over a similar period and in a very similar manner (Ödegaard 1964). His findings were surprisingly, almost disconcertingly, similar to ours both in respect to the relatively static picture following the arrival of the psychotropic drugs and to the marked change in hospital statistics during the 1940s—although in this latter phase Ödegaard identified the responsible social factor as the general fall in unemployment in Norway, which had facilitated rehabilitation. His chastening conclusion was that "in hospitals with a favorable therapeutic situation the psychotropic drugs brought little or no improvement, or even a decrease in the rate of discharges. In hospitals with a low predrug discharge rate, on the other hand, the improvement was considerable." A comparable study by Meyer et al. (1964) on case material in Munich points in the same direction.

Inasmuch as schizophrenia accounts for the bulk of long-stay mental hospital patients and has been the target for the most intensive drug therapy, it is the disorder of principal interest. A demonstration of the efficacy of treatment by epidemiological analysis depends, however, on a study of more than hopsital discharges and durations of stay. The sharp rise in the readmission rate of schizophrenics has already shown that many of them may merely have their spells in hospital converted from an uninterrupted stay to a series of fragmented episodes. For it to be shown that drugs can prevent, rather than merely delay or interrupt, hospitalization, account must be taken of extramural factors. Although this task is much more difficult because one is not dealing with a captive population, a number of attempts have been made to overcome the difficulties. Of these the most thorough and carefully designed is that of Pasamanick and his colleagues (1967), whose investigation set out to compare the two-year outcome of three different forms of treatment for identified schizophrenics. This comparison comprised (1) a control group which was treated along routine inpatient lines; (2) a group treated by prescribed doses of psychotropic drugs (chiefly phenothiazines) but maintained at home whenever possible with family support and frequent domiciliary visits by a public health nurse; and (3) a group which received identical home care but was prescribed a placebo instead of an active preparation. On the basis of their results the authors claim to have demonstrated that a substantial measure of hospitalization can be prevented by pharmacological and social measures.

It must be emphasized, nonetheless, that even if claims such as the above be substantiated—and they have not gone unchallenged—they cannot be evaluated without regard to their implications for the community services that must take responsibility for the discharged patients.

By restricting attention to such factors as cost and manpower it may appear as though unequivocal gains have been established. Such a view, however, ignores the facts, not only that most patients continue to exhibit symptoms and remain handicapped in some measure after leaving the hospital, but also that domestic conditions may be totally inadequate for a patient's extramural maintenance. Thus in Pasamanick's study the households to which the patients returned were described as "often plagued by all manner of problems: poverty, unemployment, inadequate housing, filth and squalor, marital difficulties and infidelity, problem children, insensitivity and utter callousness of family members to one another, ignorance, and physical ailments." In the United Kingdom the work of the Medical Research Council Social Psychiatry Research Unit has demonstrated clearly how necessary it is to study social attitudes and family relationships in this area (Brown et al. 1962). The careful investigation reported by Grad and Sainsbury, comparing the effects of psychiatric patients on their families in two areas—one with a hospital-based service and the other with a community care program—has demonstrated that a social price may have to be paid for the maintenance of some patients in the community (Grad and Sainsbury 1968). At present, we are very much in need of more such work so as to put clinical flesh on numerical skeletons, and so undertake a full evaluation of the place of drugs in the management of major mental disease.

REFERENCES

Brill, H., and Patton, R.E. (1959). Analysis of population reduction in New York State mental hospitals during the first four years of large-scale therapy with psychotropic drugs. *American Journal of Psychiatry* 116:495.

Brown, G.W., Monck, E.M., Carstairs, G.M., and Wing, J.K. (1962). The influence of family life on the course of schizophrenic illness. *British Journal of Preventive and Social Medicine* 16:55.

Grad, J., and Sainsbury, P. (1968). The effects that patients have on their families in a community care and control psychiatric service—a two-year follow-up. *British Journal of Psychiatry* 114:265.

Meyer, J.E., Simon, G., and Still, G. (1964). Die Therapie der Schizophrenie und der endogenen Depression zwischen 1930 und 1960. *Archiv für Psychiatrie und Nervenkrankheiten* 206:165.

Ödegaard, O. (1964). Pattern of discharge from Norwegian psychiatric hospitals before and after the introduction of the psychotropic drugs. *American Journal of Psychiatry* 120:772.

Pasamanick, B., Scarpitti, F.R., and Dinitz, S. (1967). *Schizophrenics in the Community.* New York: Appleton-Century-Crofts.

Shepherd, M., Goodman, N., and Watt, D.C. (1961). The application of hospital statistics in the evaluation of pharmacotherapy in a psychiatric population. *Comprehensive Psychiatry* 2:11.

Chapter 17

The Community Impact of Long-Acting Neuroleptics

It is now ten years since Pasamanick and his co-workers demonstrated that schizophrenic patients discharged from the hospital and subsequently maintained on oral neuroleptic drugs fared significantly better than a control group receiving placebo (Pasamanick et al. 1964). It may be recalled that the criterion which they adopted was the length of time for which the patients were able to remain out of hospital care, and in these terms their conclusions have been confirmed by subsequent work (Leff 1972). A considerable impetus to therapeutic endeavor in this direction has since been provided by the arrival of several long-acting neuroleptic drugs, most of them prescribed by injection, of which fluphenazine enanthate, fluphenazine decanoate and flupenthixol decanoate have come to be widely used.

So far, so good. It is, however, somewhat surprising to have this essentially technical advance regarded as a major innovation in the field of mental disorder. Grozier

(1973), for example, refers to it as the third revolution in psychiatry, following in the wake of Freud's contribution and the introduction of chlorpromazine by Delay and Deniker in 1952. Perhaps the case for parenteral rather than oral administration would be more compelling if this form of administration were associated with more effective pharmacodynamic action. Curry and his colleagues have provided some evidence in favor of this proposition by experiments purporting to show that chlorpromazine is metabolized and inactivated in the wall of the gastrointestinal tract, so that the injection route utilizes more available drug (Curry 1971). However, other work does not support these findings (Ravaris et al. 1965).

At the clinical level the principal evidence bearing on the efficacy of the long-term neuroleptics comes from hospital studies. As Villeneuve (1973) has said: "Currently, the main indication for the administration of a long-acting injectable neuroleptic is the maintenance treatment of schizophrenic patients who, for various reasons, do not take their oral medication and relapse." In his detailed review of the reasons for what he calls "drug deviation," Blackwell (1973) has identified several groups of factors, affecting the medication, the patient, the doctor, and the therapeutic setting, respectively. Medication factors involve the type and dosage of the drug, and side effects and length of treatment; patient reactions are determined by socioeconomic background, attitudes, and domestic circumstances; medical influences incorporate the physician's outlook, the degree of supervision, and the time elapsing since discharge from the hospital.

The identification of such factors is clearly necessary to ensure that medication is adequately ingested. What, then, are the advantages of long-term neuroleptics? Villeneuve has listed four, all of which, interestingly enough, relate to the community. The drugs, in his view: (1) enable patients to return to the community and maintain them there; (2) they ease the burden on the patients' families because drug intake is insured; (3) they facilitate the efforts of psychiatrists and of their co-workers in achieving the maximum rehabilitation of patients; and (4) they constitute an economy of time and resources.

Our local experience has some bearing on these claims. Since October 1969, four weekly clinics, in the main centers of population, have been organized to cover a population of about 450,000 in a defined area of the county of Buckinghamshire, for which St. John's Hospital, Aylesbury, provides all psychiatric services. The main purpose of the centers is to administer long-acting injected neuroleptics to schizophrenic patients living in the community. In 1973 there were 3,013 attendances at these clinics and fifty-six new patients were added during the year.

The clinics are run, and the injections administered, by one full-time, trained psychiatric nurse of St. John's Hospital, who has the part-time assistance of another nurse. Patients are reviewed regularly by referring psychiatrists, but the nurses are enabled at any time to obtain psychiatric advice, either for dosage changes, or if a patient's condition requires it. In addition to running the clinic, the nurse visits at home any patients who cannot attend, misses an appointment, or is noted as requiring attention. In 1973 about 450 home visits were made. Patients often find attendance at clinics irksome or difficult through work or domestic responsibility, and have either to be transported by a relative or have transport provided, particularly in the more rural, northern half of the county.

In order to estimate the effect of the administration of injected long-acting neuroleptic drugs under these arrangements, a follow-up of schizophrenic patients discharged from St. John's Hospital was carried out. All schizophrenics under sixty-five years of age, discharged during the years 1967-68 and 1971-2 were identified and followed up for two years subsequently, to ascertain the number of patients readmitted and the length of time spent in hospital. The first period (1968-69) precedes the establishment of the special clinics for administer ing long-term neuroleptics, while the second period (1971-72) follows it. A comparison of the follow-up data from these two periods should therefore shed some light on any effect of administering long-acting injected neuroleptics.

Table 17-1 shows, first, that significantly fewer patients were readmitted during the second period (1971-72) as compared with the first (1968-69). A further surprising finding is that, instead of being shorter, as would be expected, the average duration of stay in hospital of patients during the second period (1971-72) was longer. Table 17-2 affords an explanation of this surprising finding.

Table 17-2 shows that in the second period (1971-72) the proportion of patients not readmitted was enlarged because there was a diminution of the number of readmitted patients. However, the proportion of patients who spent more than three months in hsopital remained the same in both periods.

It is clear, therefore, that while fewer discharged schizophrenic patients were readmitted to the hospital if they were receiving long-acting neuroleptics, this advantage accrued only to those patients who, regardless of specific treatment, enjoyed a more favorable prognosis as judged by their length of stay in hospital.

It is worth considering how far the four advantages attributed by Villeneuve to the long-acting neuroleptics receive support from these findings. At first blush, the

Table 17-1

Schizophrenics readmitted within 2 years of discharge before and after institution of community administration of long-term neuroleptics.

	1967-68	1970-71
No. of schizophrenics discharged	280	244
No. of schizophrenics readmitted within 2 years*	128 (45.7%)	87 (35.7%)
Mean time spent in hospital †	145.6 days	190.7 days

$*X^2 = 5.0442$

p .05

† On median test $X^2 = 2.97$, $.05 < p < 0.1$, N.S.

findings appear to furnish evidence in favor of all four. They suggest, first, that more patients can indeed be maintained out of the hospital, in the community at large. Second, although the inquiry was not directly concerned with social factors, it relates directly to the burden shouldered by the family, inasmuch as the careful inquiry carried out by Stevens (1973) has shown that injected neuroleptics can reduce the inconvenience and

Table 17-2

Length of stay of schizophrenics readmitted to hospital within 2 years of discharge before and after institution of community administration of long-term neuroleptics.

		In Hospital		
	Not readmitted	Up to 3 mos.	More than 3 mos.	Total
1967-68	152 (54.3%)	70 (25.0%)	58 (20.7%)	280 (100%)
1970-71	157 (64.3%)	37 (15.2%)	50 (20.5%)	244 (100%)

distress occasioned by the behavior of schizophrenics at home. Third, there is no doubt that from an administrative standpoint the task of integrating doctor-nurse collaboration has been greatly facilitated and that, by the psychiatrists at least, the new arrangements have been widely accepted. There are, indeed, grounds for believing that in this area treatment by injection has come to be seen as valuable in its own right: this was most strikingly illustrated when some of the local doctors recently refused to collaborate in a double trial on the tortuous grounds that, whereas a placebo and an active drug administered by injection would be acceptable, the active drug taken orally would not. Lastly, with regard to resources, it is probably true that the long-term neuroleptic drugs have effected a saving on hospital bed occupancy, with all of its associated cost and personnel.

The above points being conceded, however, each of the seeming benefits conferred by the long-acting neuroleptic drugs must be weighed against its associated disadvantages. Thus the successful maintenance of outpatient care applies only to that half of readmitted patients whose hospital stay is shortest. Furthermore, in view of the well-recognized adverse effects of long-term neuroleptic medication, it should be emphasized that only a proportion of these patients probably require the drugs, since about one-third of a comparable population followed up by Hirsch et al. (1973) remained out of the hospital while receiving placebo alone. An additional factor to be considered is that many patients who lose the symptoms they exhibited while in the hospital can show other symptoms when at home, especially a passivity and absence of initiative which tends to render their lives rigid and uniform.

Still more important, even though the domestic problems raised by discharged schizophrenics can be relieved with drug treatment, both emotional strain and financial difficulties occur to such an extent as to indicate that the definition and measurement of these problems require social rather than clinical investigation. Two such studies carred out in the United Kingdom have underlined how, in 30-50 percent of cases, all members of the household, including children, can suffer from the return of a schizophrenic relative, even one receiving full medication (Goldberg 1971, Stevens 1972). An illustrative local case-history may be taken to demonstrate how the social repercussions can come to take precedence over the clinical phenomena:

> A twenty-six-year-old man had been discharged from hospital to live at home with his parents and a completely disabled spastic brother. When visited at home, within one year of discharge, he had returned to unskilled manual work. Although on examination he was free of overt schizophrenic symptomatology, his social life was greatly reduced. Before his illness he had been a social and active man with a keen interest in the building of motorcycles. He had completely given up this activity and never went out on his machine. He did very little at home except to watch television continuously. He felt himself to be inferior and dull and to be unable to hold a conversation with anybody. His only outside activity was to drink alcohol with his workmates at a local public house once a week.

On balance, therefore, it is evident that the patient advantages conferred by long-acting injected neuroleptic drugs must be weighed against the possible danger foreseen by the earlier American workers when they suggested that: "the mental hospital atmosphere is merely transferred to the home" (Pasamanick et al. 1964). They concluded that "An enriched program consisting of homemaking services, job-training, sheltered workshops, and more frequent access to direct psychiatric services seems to be required if the poor functioning of many 'successful' patients is to be substantially improved." Our own experience would fully confirm this view. For one thing, the handing over of aftercare from doctors to nurses can raise delicate problems of management unless medical advice is readily available. For another, from a strictly economic standpoint, the basic hospital costs can be passed on to relatives and community-services unless the patient is able to engage in gainful employment. Still more important, the process of discharge can result in the transfer of responsibility from the health service to the family, with a consequent price exacted in terms of money, health, working capacity, and the general quality of life of all concerned unless extensive support from the social services is readily accessible. All these factors must be taken into account if a realistic estimate of cost-effectiveness is to be established for the long-acting neuroleptic drugs.

In sum, then, a great deal more research remains to be undertaken before the "third revolution" in psychiatry can be assessed. Revolutions, as Lamartine pointed out, have a habit of devouring their own children, whose health and welfare would seem already to require safeguards, in the form of more extensive evaluation than has yet been undertaken.

REFERENCES

Blackwell, B. (1973). Drug deviation in psychiatric patients, In *The Future of Pharmacotherapy: New Drug Delivery Systems,* ed. F. J. Ayd, Jr., p. 17. Baltimore: International Drug Therapy Newsletter.

Curry, S. H. (1971). Chlorpromazine: concentration in plasma, excretion in urine and duration of effect. *Proceedings of the Royal Society of Medicine.* 64:285.

Goldberg, E. M. (1971). Research in social work. In *Portfolio for Health,* ed. G. Mclachlan. London: Oxford University Press.

Grozier, M. L. (1973). The third revolution in psychiatry:

fluphenazine decanoate. In *The Future of Pharmacotherapy; New Drug Delivery Systems,* ed. F. J. Ayd, Jr., p. 97. Baltimore: International Drug Therapy Newsletter.

Hirsch, S. R., Gaind, R., Rohde, P. D., Stevens, B. C., and Wing J. K. (1973). Out-patient maintenance treatment of chronic schizophrenics with fluphenazine decanoate injections: a double-blind placebo trial. *British Medical Journal* 1 633.

Leff, J. P. (1972). Maintenance therapy and schizophrenia. *British Journal of Hospital Medicine* 8:377-380.

Pasamanick, B., Scarpitt, F. R., Lefton, M., Dinitz, S., Wernent, J. J., and McPheeters, H. (1964). Home vs hospital care for schizophrenics. *Journal of the American Medical Association* 187:177-181.

Ravaris, C. L., Weaver, L. A. and Brooks, G. W. (1965). A controlled study of fluphenazine enanthate in chronic schizophrenic patients. *Diseases of the Nervous System* 26:33-39.

Stevens, B. C. (1972). Dependence of schizophrenic patients on elderly relatives. *Psychological Medicine* 2:17-32.

Stevens, B. C. (1973). The role of fluphenazine decanoate in lessening the burden of chronic schizophrenics on the community. *Psychological Medicine* 3:141-158.

Villeneuve, A. (1973). Some comments on long-acting neuroleptics. In *The Future of Pharmacotherapy: New Drug Delivery Systems,* ed. J. Ayd, Jr., p. 61. Baltimore: International Drug Therapy Newsletter.

Chapter 18

Clinical and Social Factors in the Outcome of Mental Illness

It is not always possible to define the boundaries which separate the clinical from the social aspects of disease. One useful line of demarcation runs through the methods of study: the problems which have traditionally been investigated with the techniques of the biological sciences of anatomy, physiology and pathology differ from those problems which have depended on the social sciences, particularly psychology, anthropology, and sociology. Within all disciplines, however, the focus of inquiry in the past has been on the antecedents of morbidity. But recently, there has been a quickening of interest in the consequences of established disease, which can lend themselves more readily to the study of medico-social interaction. Clear illustrations of such consequence-studies come from conditions whose etiology is indisputably exogenic. Surgical trauma constitutes an example that has lately attracted attention, especially in the United States, where the socioeconomic problems of return to work after surgery have become a matter of national concern (Dohan and Moss 1958). Through a number of inquiries into factors that determine the period of convalescence following a surgical operation, it has been demonstrated that, in addition to the metabolic responses of the body, such diverse factors as surgical folklore, the patient's motivation, and the patient's cultural attitudes to work can all influence outcome. In the fields of prosthetics and sensory disability, Meyerson has claimed that therapeutic prospects have improved since it has become appreciated that the patient's behavior depends not so much on his physical characteristics as on "the function of the situation in which the person must act" (Meyerson 1958). The extension of this viewpoint to the whole field of aftercare for physical disabilities has led to general agreement with Cooksey's (1960) proposition that "medical, psychological, social and economic factors affect the need for rehabilitation and the response to it."

The position is more complex when social and psychological factors are suspected of contributing to the etiology of physical disease, for their continued presence after the onset of illness could then be expected to prejudice its outcome. The putative relationship of occupation to coronary disease (Morris 1959) or of psychosocial factors to rheumatoid arthritis (King 1955) exemplify associations of this type, but proof still waits on a more satisfactory demonstration of the pathogenic nature of such factors than has so far proved possible. Meanwhile, there is evidence to suggest that the influence of social and psychological factors on the course of established physical illness can be studied profitably in its own right, without reference to its etiological role. In an investigation of 1630 inpatients in a general hospital, Querido (1959) has reported on the forecasts made by clinicians and by an independent team consisting of a social worker and a psychiatrist who concentrated on "the social and/or psychic conditions which impair. . . well-being." The patients were followed up for six months and it was found that, irrespective of physical diagnosis, recovery was significantly less frequent among the "distressed" patients, even though the nature of their distress did not appear to be specific. Furthermore, the predictions of recovery made by the social worker/psychiatrist team were significantly more accurate than those based on clinical considerations alone. The clinical value of this work would be greater, if it were refined in relations to individual disorders (Gainsborough and Slater 1946). Our own preliminary findings with selected conditions, however, are less clear-cut.

The place of psychosocial factors in the background and outcome of the major psychiatric disorders is widely recognized; it is functionally acknowledged by the empirical but indispensable role of the psychiatric social worker in the management of these conditions. In theory, the interplay of social and clinical factors on the course of psychiatric illness can be studied along lines similar to those which obtain in physical disease; in practice, this exercise often proves to be most fruitful when the diagnostic concepts are most sharply defined and the social issues are least obscure. Thus, the outcome of an organic dementia may obviously depend as much on the patient's socioeconomic status, and on the tolerance of his relatives, as on the degree of his disability.

The application of more sophisticated sociological concepts to psychiatric illness is in its early stages (Clausen 1959). Most of this work has been concerned with etiology, but its relevance to outcome is clearly demonstrated in the sphere of mental subnormality, where the ease of case-identification and the subject's contact with social agencies have facilitated several long-term follow-up studies over many years. On the basis of these results it has been noted that the mentally subnormal do better than might be suggested by the medicosocial evidence covering their early years (Charles 1953, National Committee for Mental Hygiene 1933). Among the factors which might contribute to these findings, Stein and Susser have recently selected and studied certain features of the family group (Stein and Susser 1960). Drawing on social and anthropological theory, these workers have classified families into "functioning," "deviant," and "dysmorphic" units according to their ability to provide, first, "a set of enduring human relationships" and secondly, "basic standards of care for the children." In a sample of children ascertained as educationally subnormal and later examined in early adult life, Stein and Susser were able to demonstrate how closely their family groupings could be related to their outcome in terms of domestic stability, employment record, contacts with the law, and admissions to institutions. They have suggested also that seeming increments of intelligence among defective subjects without brain injury may be related to familial subcultures classified by occupational and educational criteria.

The functional psychoses raise problems of their own. The numerous follow-up studies on these conditions have for the most part been conducted within the Kraepelinian framework, and have tended to incorporate outcome as an axis for diagnostic classification. The authors of a recent study have put the matter squarely: "as long as the etiology and pathogenesis of the schizophrenic disorders are unknown the diagnosis and differential diagnosis of schizophrenia must be based upon an analysis of the clinical symptoms and an evaluation of the outcome of the disease" (Holmboe and Astrup 1957). Accordingly, the aim of most of these inquiries has been the analysis of clinical data which might facilitate and improve the *Richtungsprognose* of the older clinicians. Outcome has been defined in several ways, including the length of illness, the recurrence of attacks, the present or absence of defect states, and the chances of acquiring an hereditary disorder. These questions have been related primarily to such clinical features as abruptness of onset, the occurrence of particular symptoms, the premorbid personality, and the body build. By contrast, social factors have been so neglected in this universe of studies that Langfeldt has concluded that nothing of much significance has been stated as to the influence of psychological and social factors on the course of schizophrenia (Langfeldt 1959).

But however firmly clinical investigators have inclined to such a view they have been unable to sustain it when considering the problems of therapy. The treatment of the functional psychoses has necessitated an interest in psychosocial factors from two standpoints. The first has been the direct influence of these factors on the outcome of the disease. In this field the careful studies of the Medical Research Council Social Psychiatry Unit into the effects of artificial incentives (Topping and O'Conner 1960), hospital workshops (Carstairs et al. 1956), industrial rehabilitation centers (Wing 1960), and domestic conditions (Brown 1959) on the course of chronic schizophrenia may be cited as illustrations of the Unit's director's maxim that "rehabilitation is treatment from the social point of view" (Lewis 1956).

The other aspect of therapeutics that has implicated social factors in the outcome of the functional psychoses is the need to develop criteria for the evaluation of their treatment. Explicitly or implicitly, clinicians have been compelled to pay regard to the social dimension in describing the outcome of the functional psychoses. Many psychiatrists have been content with imprecise yardsticks such as "social recovery" or "social remission." Most of the attempts to refine such criteria have been related principally to schizophrenia, although, as Lundquist has emphasized, the social consequences of the manic depressive psychoses also repay attention (Lundquist 1945). Twenty years ago Guttmann, Mayer-Gross and Slater proposed a scale of responses to therapy which passed from "total recovery" to "social recovery," "social defect," "family invalidism," and "hospital invalidism" (Guttmann et al. 1939). In Great Britain these criteria have been used unchanged by other workers (Leiberman et al. 1957). Elsewhere, authorities like Delay accept a triple standard of "hospital improvement," "social improvement," and "complete remission of symptoms" (Delay et al. 1959). Bleuler subdivides both schizophrenic deterioration and recovery into "social" and "complete" (Bleuler 1955); and Max Müller has suggested that a full *restitutio ad integrum* could be regarded as no more than "a good social remission" (Muller 1949).

Our own interest in these factors some years ago prompted a study of 126 patients who had suffered acute schizophrenic illnesses for which they had been treated by deep insulin coma therapy (Shepherd 1959). In following up these patients for five years we were primarily concerned with studying clinical and social indices of outcome and the relationships between these. In brief, we found that the presence of the major schizophrenic phenomena and a long stay in hospital went closely with the patients' dependence on external support, a poor work-record, and an unsatisfactory set of relatives' attitudes. We also found that only one clinical symptom, deterioration of affect, was associated with a poor medico social outcome. On the other hand, any symptoms or behavior that were considered embarrassing or dangerous affected the outcome adversely, partly by increasing the time spent in hospital, and partly by dissuading relatives from accepting responsibility for the patient.

We also collected data bearing on the social mobility of these patients and their parents, noting that there was an inter-generation decline when the parents belonged to social classes 1 and 2, but not when they were placed in social classes 4 or 5. Observations of this type, as Firth has pointed out, indicate where to look for further information but do not tell us what to look for (Firth 1958). In a recent study of the bearing of social class on the prognosis in schizophrenia, Cooper has examined the question of social mobility in more detail (Cooper 1961). Finding that patients from the upper social classes enjoyed a more favorable outcome than did those from the lower social groups, he studied the social histories of 192 male schizophrenics after their first stay in hospital. Although the patients' clinical condition at discharge was unrelated to their social status, their subsequent occupational histories differed significantly by social class. Cooper's results support the view that the higher the patient's social status the better was his chance of maintaining it. They also show that a majority of patients who were unable to maintain their previous occupational level were unable to work at all. The trend towards downward social mobility was most marked in the lower social groups but was insufficient to account for the observed social gradient, and on the basis of his data Cooper has suggested that the differential outcome is linked most closely to the increased socioeconomic stress which confronts those patients who are less cushioned in the economic struggle and who have fewer skills on which to fall back.

Occupational adaptation has also figured prominently in the follow-up studies of patients suffering from the neuroses and personality disorders (Lewis 1943, Ernst 1959). Clinical practice shows this group of conditions to be so frequently embedded in, and often dependent on, a matrix of social and interpersonal disturbances that our lack of precise knowledge about the influence of psychosocial factors on their outcome constitutes a major challenge to future investigators. One of the principal obstacles in the way of adequate studies has been the practical problem of tracing groups of people who are notoriously elusive. For this reason captive populations, such as military personnel, tend to provide opportunities that remain attractive despite their obvious limitations (Guttmann and Thomas 1946). Perhaps the most striking demonstration of a successfully prosecuted study of this type has been provided by the five-year follow-up of 1,475 randomly selected American soldiers in World War II, with a control group of several hundred enlisted men (Brill and Beebe 1955). It emerged that, contrary to expectation, the general trend toward improvement among the men who had been discharged with a neurotic disability was related to their subsequent social circumstances rather than to their military experiences, the degree of their disability, or the treatment they received. Brill and Beebe's findings led them toward a detailed consideration of their subjects' socio economic milieu and away from the niceties of their individual psychology. This trend has become increasingly pronounced in comparable civilian investigations, where the spur has been chiefly an interest in the evaluation of psychotherapy. For this purpose, Miles et al. have argued that the rounded picture must include not only clinical symptoms but a separate assessment of social adjustment in terms of occupational record, interpersonal relations, marital and sexual harmony (Miles et al. 1951). So far, very few workers have succeeded in adopting this approach, but its potential value was demonstrated by one of our follow-up studies of alcoholics, most of whom were suffering from neurotic or personality disorders of some kind (Shepherd 1957). Here a prognostic formulation in terms of particular symptoms—in this case consumption of alcohol—carried less meaning than a formulation which took the patient's functional capacity into account. Our profile of the patient with a favorable outcome, for example, was as follows: "an intermittent drinker of good previous personality, with a satisfactory work-record, with close personal ties to at least some one person, married, seeking help for the first time, rating I for social stability, anxious to accept the aid of disulfiram and Alcoholics Anonymous." In this composite picture, made up only of those items related to outcome, the significance of social features is evident.

A prime methodological defect in the great majority of studies bearing on the outcome of neurosis has been their dependence on the hospital patient. Since only a small proportion of such patients may be referred to hospitals other techniques must be developed if more representative groups are to be examined. Scandinavian researchers have, for example, taken advantage of their circumscribed communities and their admirable population statistics. In Great Britain the general practitioners offer a promising lead. Whatever the method employed, however, it is now apparent that in the study of minor psychiatric illnesses in the community, clinicans will require the help of their colleagues from the social sciences to study the environment in which patients with these illnesses live and through which they often express their symptoms. From such collaborative studies we can hope to acquire a better understanding of these conditions in terms of John Ryle's distinction between the natural history of disease in man and the natural history of man in disease.

REFERENCES

Bleuler, M. (1955). Reasearch and changes in concepts in the study of schizophrenia, 1941-50. *Bulletin of the Isaac Ray Medical Library* 3:1.

Brill, N.Q., and Beebe, G.W. (1955). *A Follow-up Study of War Neuroses.* Washington: United States Government Printing Office.

Brown, G.W. (1959). Experiences of discharged chronic schizophrenic patients in various types of living groups. *Milbank Memorial Fund Quarterly* 37:105.

Carstairs, G.M., O'Connor, N., and Rawnsley, K. (1956). Organisation of a hospital workshop for chronic psychotic patients. *British Journal of Preventive and Social Medicine*: 10:136.

Charles, D.C. (1953). Ability and accomplishment of persons earlier judged mentally deficient. *Genetic Psychology Monographs* 47:3.

Clausen, J.A. (1959). The sociology of mental illness. In *Sociology Today,* ed. R.K. Merton, L. Broom, and L.S. Cottrell. N.Y.: Basic.

Conference on surgical convalescence. *Annals of the New York Academy of Sciences* 73:38, 1958.

Cooksey, F.S. (1960). Progress and problems in the rehabilitation of disabled people. *Proceedings of the Royal Society of Medicine* 53:707.

Cooper, A.B. (1961). Social class and prognosis in schizophrenia. *Journal of Preventive and Social Medicine* 15:17.

Delay, J., Deniker, P., and Ropert, R. (1959). The place of neuroleptic chemotherapy in treatment of schizophrenic states. In *Psychopharmacology Frontiers,* ed. N.S. Kline, p. 105. Boston, Little, Brown and Company, Inc.

Ernst, K. (1959). *Die Prognose der Neurosen.* Monographien aus dem Gesamtgebeite der Neurologie und Psychiatrie, Number 85. Berlin: Springer.

Firth, R. (1958). Habits and ways of life in relation to the development of chronic disease, p. 83. In *Symposium on the Public Health Aspects of Chronic Disease,* p. 83. Copenhagen: World Health Organization.

Gainsborough, H., and Slater, E. T. O. (1946). A study of peptic ulcer. *British Medical Journal* 2:253.

Guttmann, E., Mayer-Gross, W., and Slater, E.T.O. (1939). Short distance prognosis of schizophrenia. *Journal of Neurology, Neurosurgery and Psychiatry* 25:266.

Guttmann, E., and Thomas, E.L. (1946). *A Report on the Readjustment in Civil Life of Soldiers Discharged from the Army on Account of Neurosis.* Reports on Public Health Medical Subjects, Number 93. London: H.M.S.O.

Holmboe, R., and Astrup, C. (1957). A follow-up study of 255 patients with acute schizophrenia and schizophreniform psychoses. *Acta Psychiatrica et Neurologica , Supplement* 115. Copenhagen: Munksgaard.

King, S.H. (1955). Psychosocial factors associated with rheumatoid arthritis. *Journal of Chronic Diseases* 2:287.

Langfeldt, G. (1959). *The Prognosis in Schizophrenia.* Vol. 1. 2nd International Congress for Psychiatry, ed. W.A. Stoll. Zurich: p. 220.

Leiberman, D.M., Hönig, J. and Auerbach, I. (1957). The effect of insulin coma and ECT on the 3-year prognosis of schizophrenia. *Journal of Neurology, Neurosurgery and Psychiatry* 20:108.

Lewis, A. (1943). Social Effects of Neurosis. *Lancet* 1:167.

Lewis, A. (1956). Rehabilitation programmes in England. In *The Elements of a Community Mental Health Programme,* p. 196. New York: Milbank Memorial Fund.

Lundquist, G. (1945). Prognosis and course in manic-depressive psychoses. *Acta Psychiatrica et Neurologica, Supplement XXXV.* Stockholm.

Meyerson, L. (1958). Psychological aspects of sensory disability. *Annals of the New York Academy of Sciences* 74:128.

Miles, M.H.W., Barrabee, E.L., and Finesinger, J.E. (1951). Evaluation of psychotherapy. *Psychosomatic Medicine* 13:83.

Morris, J.N. (1959). Occupation and coronary heart disease. *Archives of Internal Medicine* 104:903.

Muller, M. (1949). *Prognose und Therapie der Geisteskrankheiten.* Stuttgart: Georg Thieme.

National Committee for Mental Hygiene (1933). The subnormal child—17 years later. *Mental Hygiene* 17:177.

Querido, A. (1959). Forecast and follow-up. *British Journal of Preventive and Social Medicine* 13:33.

Shepherd, M. (1957). Alcoholism: A medical and social problem. *Medical World* 87:246.

Shepherd, M. (1959). The social outcome of early schizophrenia. *Psychiatrica et Neurologica* 137:224.

Stein, Z., and Susser, M. (1960). The families of dull children. *British Journal of Preventive and Social Medicine* 14, 83: and *Journal of Mental Science* 106:1296, 1304 and 1311.

Topping, G.G., and O'Connor, N. (1960). The response of chronic schizophrenics to incentives. *British Journal of Medical Psychology* 33:211.

Wing, J.K (1960). Pilot experiment in the rehabilitation of long-hospitalized male schizophrenic patients. *British Journal of Preventive and Social and Medicine* 14:173.

Epilogue

Chapter 19

A View in Prospect

The foundations of clinical psychiatry as we know it today were laid principally by European clinicians, persons whose training and professional activities were focused on diagnosis and treatment. The energy, purpose, and skill which these pioneers brought to their refractory material resulted in the descriptive mapping of the major forms of mental disorder which necessitate institutional care. Their impressive achievement can be attributed to the notion of the clinician functioning as his own research instrument, which led to an insistence on careful clinical observation as the bedrock of the discipline. It also led, however, to the propounding of ambitious claims on behalf of the clinical method, of which the following—advanced by an eminent clinician at the First International Congress of Psychiatry in 1950—is an example:

> Clinical psychiatry is the firm center of scientific psychiatry. . . . Today in my opinion the signature of clinical

> psychiatry is that all the currents which made their appearance separately in the history of the ages, either paying attention exclusively to the physical or exclusively to the somatic aspect, or solely to philosophical penetration, or above all, to pure empiricism, or understanding while ignoring ethics, or understanding only from deviations from ethics, are now led by the clinician into one channel in one great theory, encompassing them all. [Rumke 1950]

With hindsight we must, in my view, take a much less inflated view of the clinical psychiatrist's function in research. In this regard it is instructive to recall that in the field of internal medicine, the growth of clinical science in the past two generations has so eroded the former authority of the clinician as to have stimulated a recent, spirited defense of clinical judgment—with one basic proviso: "The clinician can organize, classify, process and analyze his data with exactly the same intellectual, statistical, and computational procedures available in every other branch of science. For these procedures to yield valuable scientific results, however, the clinician must also improve the scientific validity of the primary clinical data" (Feinstein 1967).

In too many quarters this warning has been least heeded in psychiatry, where we have paid the price for self-indulgent complacency, the payment having been exacted in terms of an excessive preoccupation with the minutiae of symptomatology and with sterile arguments about classification more reminiscent of medieval schools of theology than of modern schools of medicine. On this topic academic pronouncements have been made in such terms as to recall Nietzsche's comment to Burckhardt that he "would very much prefer a professorial chair in Basel to being God." Challenges to such an attitude have, nonetheless, been proclaimed in the form of evidence from at least three sources, which make it clear that the clinical psychiatrists should be prepared to exercise more modesty than he has been wont to do in the past. Work in these three areas questions the traditional authority of the clinician with respect to his diagnostic competence, his therapeutic skills, and his familiarity with the full spectrum of clinical issues comprehended by his specialty.

CHALLENGES TO THE CLINICIAN

The first challenge to the psychiatric clinician comes from careful scrutiny of the subjective nature of many of the data used in the classical descriptions of mental illness. Some of the fallacies inherent in an over dependence on this category of information were exposed in the international study of observer variation, carried out for the World Health Organization in the form of an experimental approach to psychiatric diagnosis (Shepherd et al. 1968). In this study, the use of standardized case histories and videotaped interviews revealed disconcertingly large areas of disagreement between a group of experts from several countries, and showed clearly that there are marked variations in the observations and perceptions of the most experienced clinicians, in the clinical inferences drawn from clinical data, and in the classificatory schemata in use at the present time. It is becoming widely accepted that clinical psychiatry sorely lacks not only an acceptable schema of classification but also an accompanying glossary of terms, a task to which the World Health Organization is addressing itself at the present time.

The second challenge to the clinician arises from the field of experimental therapeutics. In every branch of medicine the pharmacologist and the medical statistician can now supplement, and often contradict, the authoritative pronouncements of clinical experience with expert knowledge not only of the principles of pharmaco-dynamics but also of experimental design. Nowhere is such expertise more essential than in psychiatry, where a paucity of objective indices renders measurement difficult and clinical impressions treacherous. The importance of this point of view has been amply demonstrated by the development of a peculiarly British contribution to clinical methodology—the controlled clinical trial. This form of clinical experiment was largely developed in the 1930s by the Clinical Trials Committee of the Medical Research Council under the guidance of Professor Sir Austin Bradford Hill. Accordingly, when the Medical Research Council extended its activities to cover mental disease some ten years ago, the evaluation of remedies for mental disorder may be said to have come of age. The possibilities of the controlled clinical trial were well illustrated by the first study conducted under this aegis, a large-scale, multicentered evaluation of four treatments of depressive illnesses—electric shock, two drugs, and a placebo—in which 250 patients were treated and followed up for six months by fifty-five psychiatrists working in thirty different hospitals (Medical Research Council Clinical Psychiatry Committee 1965). The theoretical justification for so elaborate an investigation resides in the need to obtain and study a homogeneous cohort of patients much larger than an individual clinician, or group of clinicians, can reasonably hope to amass. In this instance the practical justification proved to reside in unexpected results which confounded clinical opinion about therapeutic response and the efficacy of treatment.

The third challenge to the clinician is posed by the application of epidemiological principles to the study of mental disorders. It is now apparent that hospital-based psychiatrists have generalized about these disorders from what the statistically-minded critic would recognize as a grossly unrepresentative sample. For example, studies of mental illness in general practice in the United Kingdon have shown that the nature and distribution of psychiatric morbidity are very different from what is encountered in hospital practice and, still more to the point, that not more than one in twenty of these patients are referred to any form of hospital facility (Shepherd et al. 1966). We are only now beginning to take cognizance of the full range of extramural mental illness as part of a deepening interest in community medicine. Furthermore, the emphasis being placed on early discharge and community care has revealed that many of the phenomena of major mental disease have to be regarded as institutionally determined artifacts which can be modified by energetic intervention.

COGNATE DISCIPLINES

But while the formal application of the scientific method to the clinical data of psychiatry holds out great promise for the future, it is equally evident that, as with other branches of medicine, clinical research in psychiatry must also incorporate the concepts and findings of cognate disciplines. For even so perceptive a clinician as Emil Kraepelin the disciplines in question were wholly identified with the biological sciences: "Clinical observation," he wrote, "must be supplemented by thorough examination of healthy and diseased brains, neurology, the study of heredity and degenerative diseases, the chemistry of metabolism and serology" (Kraepelin 1962). The laboratory studies which established the neurosyphilitic basis of general paresis, or the metabolic investigations of Gjessing on periodic catatonia, can be accounted successful examples of research in this mold, but it is historically significant that even before Kraepelin expressed these views there had appeared the first group of the remarkable series of papers by Joseph Goldberger which were to demonstrate the dietary etiology of pellegra and its associated psychiatric disorders by means of a purely epidemiological analysis (Terris 1964). Nor is it entirely fanciful to assume, in the light of the clinical knowledge which had been amassed about general paresis by the second half of the nineteenth century, that an epidemiologist of Goldberger's ability could have established that syphilis was a necessary link in the etiological chain long before Wassermann and Noguchi had clinched the case.

Clearly Kraepelin's list of the basic sciences relevant to psychiatry must be regarded as incomplete. The experience of the past fifty years has now confirmed that these sciences are broadly divisible into two large categories: the biological group, which includes neuroanatomy, neurophysiology, neuroendocrinology, ethology, neurochemistry, and pharmacology; and the psychosocial group, which includes psychology, sociology, anthropology, and demography. Psychology is a bridging discipline between these groups: on the one hand it extends into the indisputably nonbiological areas of social and educational psychology; on the other hand, the techniques of modern neuropsychology are often closer to physiology than to psychology in the traditional sense. In general, the psychosocial sciences are concerned with the identification of factors bearing on the causal associations and natural history of mental diseases, while the biological sciences are concerned with the mechanisms and interactions of such factors. In this respect, of course, the subject does not differ essentially from general medicine, where the situation has been well described in the form of an extended metaphor:

> Medicine is at heart a polygamist becoming wedded to as many of the sciences and practial arts as prove their worth.

> . . . As is often the case with polygamy, the first set of wives—say, the biological and chemical sciences—are reluctant at first to approve yet another addition to the menage. But there is still hope. As the burden of work plainly becomes more than can be managed by the present members of the household, they become ready for new accessions to help carry the load of what needs to be done. [Merton 1957]

DEPENDENCE ON ALLIED SCIENCES

The complexity of the network of scientific disciplines which may contribute to progress in psychiatry emerges from any survey of recent advances in knowledge. To mention, for example, no more than human genetics, the neurochemistry of inborn errors of metabolism, learning theory, or the development of the new psychotropic drugs is to indicate the dependence of modern psychiatry on a host of allied sciences. It follows that scientific research in the field of mental disorders must depend not only on the independent contributions of workers in a number of related disciplines, but also on the interchange between such workers and clinicians. It therefore becomes imperative to provide the research-minded psychiatrist with easy access to other workers in related fields of research for a simple but good reason: "When psychiatrists are closely in touch with people conducting research in other medical or scientific fields, and are not isolated in groups wholly engaged in clinical routine, and when they are men whose training and interests are of a kind to make them ready to consider new information and to see old information in a new light, the chances that a train of discovery will be fired are high" (Lewis 1963).

At the present time the numbers involved are still pitifully small. Indeed, it has been estimated that research is the primary activity of no more than about forty psychiatrists in the United Kingdom (Vickers 1968).

With so much to do and so few people available it would seem reasonable to assume that any large-scale program of psychiatric research will take some time to develop. This being the case, the problem of priorities must inevitably arise, and so it is of some interest to recall that five years ago a W.H.O. Scientific Group in Mental Health Research not only surveyed research needs but estimated their relative priority for W.H.O. action. Naturally the aims of an international body must differ in many respects from those of any national group, but the considered opinion of a group of experts must carry some weight in considering research strategy. In descending order of priority the listed topics were: (1) epidemiology and social psychiatry; (2) the study of cultural and environmental factors; (3) the genetics of mental disorder; (4) mental retardation; (5) studies of childhood development; (6) geriatric psychiatry; (7) the application of learning theory; (8) biological psychiatry; (9) psychosomatic disorders; (10) psychotherapy; (11) alcoholism and drug abuse; (12) industrial psychiatry; and (13) forensic psychiatry. The study of psychotropic drugs will enter into several of these areas of investigation.

REFERENCES

Feinstein, A.R. (1967). *Clinical Judgment*. Baltimore: Williams and Wilkins, p. 287.

Kraepelin, E. (1962). *One Hundred Years of Psychiatry*. Trans. Wade Baskin, p. 152. New York: Citadel.

Lewis, A. (1963). *Research and its Application in Psychiatry*. Glasgow: Jackson, p. 20.

Medical Research Council Clinical Psychiatry Committee (1965). Clinical trial of the treatment of depressive illness. *British Medical Journal* 1:881.

Medical Research Council (1968a). *Annual Report, April 1967-March 1968,* p. 185. London: Her Majesty's Stationery Office.

Merton, R.K. (1957). Some preliminaries to a sociology of medical education. In: *The Student-Physician,* ed. R.K. Merton, G.G. Reader, and P.L. Kendall, p. 32. Cambridge, Mass.: Harvard University Press.

Rumke, H.C. (1950). In *Psychopathologie Generale, Congres International de Psychiatrie.* Vol. 1. Paris: Hermann, p. 174.

Shepherd, M., Brooke, E.M., Cooper, J.E., and Lin, T.Y. (1968). *Acta Psychiatrica Scandinavica* 44: Supplement Number 201.

Shepherd, M., Cooper, B., Brown, A.C., and Kalton, G.W. (1966). *Psychiatric Illness in General Practice.* London: Oxford, p. 159.

Terris, M. (ed.) (1964). *Goldberger on Pellagra.* Baton Rouge: Louisiana State University Press.

Vickers, G. (1968). The promotion of psychiatric research. *British Journal of Psychiatry* 114: 925.

Index